ERGONOMICS IN BACK PAIN

A Guide to Prevention and Rehabilitation

ERGONOMICS IN BACK PAIN

A Guide to Prevention and Rehabilitation

Tarek M. Khalil, Ph.D., P.E.
Elsayed M. Abdel-Moty, Ph.D.
Renee S. Rosomoff, R.N., M.B.A., C.R.N.
Hubert L. Rosomoff, M.D., D. Med. Sc.

VNR VAN NOSTRAND REINHOLD
_____ New York

Copyright © 1993 by Van Nostrand Reinhold

Library of Congress Catalog Card Number 93-1589
ISBN 0-442-01375-2

All rights reserved. No part of this work covered by the copyright hereon may be reproduced or used in any form or by any means—graphic, electronic, or mechanical, including photocopying, recording, taping, or information storage and retrieval systems—without written permission of the publisher.

I(T)P Van Nostrand Reinhold is a division of International Thomson Publishing. ITP logo is a trademark under license.

Printed in the United States of America.

Van Nostrand Reinhold
115 Fifth Avenue
New York, New York 10003

International Thomson Publishing
Berkshire House
168–173 High Holborn
London WC1V 7AA, England

Thomas Nelson Australia
102 Dodds Street
South Melbourne 3205
Victoria, Australia

Nelson Canada
1120 Birchmount Road
Scarborough, Ontario M1K 5G4, Canada

16 15 14 13 12 11 10 9 8 7 6 5 4 3 2 1

Library of Congress Cataloging-in-Publication Data

Ergonomics in back pain : a guide to prevention and rehabilitation / Tarek M. Khalil . . . [et al.].
    p.   cm.
    Includes bibliographical references and index.
    ISBN 0-442-01375-2
    1. Backache—Prevention. 2. Backache—Treatment. 3. Human engineering. I. Khalil, Tarek M.
RD771.B217E74   1993
617.5'64—dc20
                                      93-1589
                                          CIP

Preface

The study, analysis, prevention, and rehabilitation of musculoskeletal injuries is an ongoing challenge to ergonomists, safety specialists, and health care delivery practitioners. One area of particular interest is low back pain. The introduction of ergonomics to the rehabilitation and management of pain patients represents a new horizon for ergonomic research and application in a much needed area. This book is written to address the contributions that ergonomics can offer in this regard.

Chapter 1 of this book introduces ergonomics to the reader through definitions, basic concepts, and the scope of this science. The value of using ergonomic principles to study the interaction between people and their work or living environment is demonstrated through a description of the human-machine system. The concept of stress as a demand placed by the environment on the human body is presented and followed as a theme throughout the discussion of the various topics. The importance of studying the human system in relation to the workplace is addressed through practical examples.

Chapter 2 addresses the magnitude of the problem of low back pain. Epidemiologic data are presented. Figures showing the devastating effects of low back pain on the economy, industry, lost work days, and health care delivery are given. The origins of low back pain and the events leading to injury are tabulated. Causes of back pain and their effects on functional disability are presented with specific reference to occupational factors.

Chapter 3 presents the role of ergonomics in the management of low back pain at the three stages: pre-injury, rehabilitation, and post-rehabilitation. The role of the medical community in the evaluation and treatment of low back pain is summarized and the contributions of the ergonomist in a multidisciplinary health care delivery team are explained.

In Chapters 4 through 10, intervention strategies are presented. The ergonomic approach to human performance analysis and functional capacity assessment as well as measurement methods is discussed. Other intervention strategies that deal with the problem of functional disability resulting from low back pain are presented. The scientific concepts and value of using electromyography, muscle reeducation, biomechanics, biofeedback, and functional electric stimulation in the management of low back pain are given. Intervention through workplace design and analysis are detailed. The different principles, methods, and practical considerations of workplace design are discussed.

Chapter 11 provides the reader with examples of ergonomic interventions in the reengineering of workplaces and job tasks to minimize stresses and improve productivity. Case studies and population profiles are drawn from actual applications at the Comprehensive Pain and Rehabilitation Center of the University of Miami.

Several appendices provide the reader with constants, conversion factors, forms, and other useful information needed in ergonomic work. The book is written with the idea that it can be used by the many disciplines dealing with back pain and musculoskeletal problems in general, including ergonomists, physicians, physical therapists, occupational therapists, counselors, chiropractors, doctors of osteopathic medicine, as well as rehabilitation specialists.

It is hoped that this book can serve as a point of light in the quest to relieve the millions of back pain and musculoskeletal injury sufferers of their problems.

Contents

Chapter 1   **Ergonomics: Definition and Scope**   1

                      THE BASIS OF THE ERGONOMIC APPROACH   3

Chapter 2   **Low Back Pain**   8

                      THE PAIN SENSATION   8
                      PREVALENCE OF LOW BACK PAIN   9
                      LOW BACK PAIN IN THE WORKPLACE   11
                      COST OF THE LOW BACK PAIN PROBLEM   12
                      STRUCTURE OF THE BACK   14
                      ORIGINS OF LOW BACK PAIN   23
                      RISK FACTOR   28
                      ACUTE VERSUS CHRONIC PAIN   31
                      THE CYCLES OF PAIN   32
                      THE DISABILITY, IMPAIRMENT, AND
                          DYSFUNCTION OF LOW BACK PAIN
                          PATIENTS   33

Chapter 3   **Low Back Pain Management and the Role of Ergonomics**   35

                      ERGONOMICS IN THE PRE-INJURY STAGE   36
                      THE POST-INJURY REHABILITATION
                          STAGE   37
                      ERGONOMICS IN THE POST-INJURY
                          REHABILITATION STAGE   48

ERGONOMICS IN THE POST-REHABILITATION
  STAGE 52
METHODS OF ERGONOMIC
  INTERVENTIONS 53

Chapter 4 **Principles and Methods of Ergonomic Job Analysis and Workplace Design 55**

METHODS OF ERGONOMIC JOB ANALYSIS 56
ANALYSIS OF THE SITTING WORKPLACE 58
WORKING WITH VISUAL DISPLAY
  TERMINALS 62
COMPUTER-AIDED WORKPLACE DESIGN 66
GENERAL GUIDELINES FOR WORKPLACE
  DESIGN 72

Chapter 5 **Principles and Methods of Interventions Through Postural Correction 73**

ANATOMICAL PLANES OF REFERENCE 73
POSTURE AND HEALTH 74
PRINCIPLES RELATED TO POSTURE 79
POSTURE AND ENERGY DEMAND 81

Chapter 6 **Principles and Methods of Interventions Through Biomechanical Approaches to Stress Reduction 87**

THE LEVER SYSTEM ACTION 87
MECHANICAL ADVANTAGES OF LEVERS 89
BIOMECHANICAL MODELS 89

Chapter 7 **Principles and Methods of Interventions Through Knowledge and Awareness of Body Mechanics 94**

COMPATIBLE AND NONCOMPATIBLE
  MOVEMENTS 94
BODY MECHANICS IN LIFTING 95

Chapter 8   **Principles and Methods of Interventions Through the Evaluation of Human Characteristics**   **101**

    COMPONENTS OF THE HUMAN PERFORMANCE PROFILE   106
    EVALUATION OF PEOPLE WITH CHRONIC PAIN OR INJURY   140

Chapter 9   **Principles and Methods of Interventions Through Biofeedback, Muscle Reeducation, and Functional Electric Stimulation**   **147**

    BIOFEEDBACK   147
    MUSCLE REEDUCATION   149
    FUNCTIONAL ELECTRICAL STIMULATION   149

Chapter 10   **Principles and Methods of Interventions Through Work Conditioning and Work Hardening**   **152**

    WORK CONDITIONING   152
    WORK HARDENING   153

Chapter 11   **Applications and Case Studies of Erogonmic Interventions**   **154**

    CASE STUDIES IN ERGONOMIC JOB ANALYSIS, POSTURE, AND BODY MECHANICS   154
    BIOMECHANICS   167
    EVALUATION OF HUMAN CHARACTERISTICS   169
    ELECTROMYOGRAPHY   174
    PHYSICAL CONDITIONING   182

Appendix A   **Conversion Factors**   **208**

Appendix B Constants and Multipliers   213

Appendix C Definitions and Formulas   214

Appendix D Body Weight Segments   217

Appendix E Key To Job Demands   218

Index   219

Table of Abbreviations

ADA	Americans with Disabilities Act
ADL	activities of daily living
AMA	American Medical Association
AME	acceptable maximum effort
BW	band width
CLBP	chronic low back pain
CNS	central nervous system
CPRC	Comprehensive Pain and Rehabilitation Center
CT	computer-assisted tomography
DOL	Department of Labor
DOT	Dictionary of Occupational Titles
EJA	ergonomic job analysis
EMG	electromyography
FCA	functional capacity assessment
FES	functional electric stimulation
FRI	functional restoration index
FWRI	full-wave rectified integral
HMS	human-machine system
HPP	human performance profile
Hz	hertz
lb	pound
LB	low back
LBP	low back pain
LSA	lumbosacral angle
MAW	maximum acceptable weight
MDW	maximum dynamic weight
MPS	myofascial pain syndrome
MRI	magnetic resonance imaging
msec	milliseconds

MVC	maximum voluntary contraction
NIOSH	National Institute of Occupational Safety & Health
OT	occupational therapy
PT	physical therapy
RFC	residual functional capacity
RMS	root mean square value
ROM	ranges of motion
SI	sacroiliac
uV	microvolts
VDT	visual display terminals

ERGONOMICS IN BACK PAIN

A Guide to Prevention and Rehabilitation

1
Ergonomics: Definition and Scope

The term *ergonomics* is derived from two Greek words: ergon meaning work, and nomos meaning natural laws. Ergonomics is the scientific study of people and their work. The study of people includes their characteristics, customs, habits, and limitations. These limitations may be because of structure, function, or behavior. People's work includes physical or mental activities undertaken in the process of daily living or in the pursuit of achieving a goal such as producing a product, delivering a service, or engaging in a leisure activity. The study of work also entails the tools, equipment, and ambient environment in which work activities are performed. These are usually referred to in the ergonomic literature as the *work environment*.

A major premise of ergonomics is that people have certain recognizable characteristics and it is always possible to design the task, the equipment, and the environment to be compatible with those characteristics. The principle involved is that providing a good match between people and their environment can result in better human performance, as well as in the enhancement of health and safety. The design concept that centers around this principle is called *human-centered design*, which recognizes that the focus of every designed system must be the human being.

Ergonomic principles are valuable in improving the quality of life, and their application spans all human related activities. The use of ergonomics is relevant in every type and size of organization.

Ergonomics is highly relevant to preventive and occupational medicine, the management of musculoskeletal injuries, and rehabilitation. Ergonomics helps people understand their abilities and limitations and teaches them how to perform safely, effectively, and comfortably within the environment. In fact, when applied to the medical and rehabilitation fields, ergonomics has a

2 Ergonomics in Back Pain

distinct advantage over all other scientific fields. It contributes to the prevention of injuries (primary prevention), to the rehabilitation and management of trauma and health disorders (secondary prevention), and to the post-rehabilitation stage (tertiary prevention), where the return to a productive lifestyle and the reduction of stresses, with the goal of reducing chances of reinjury, becomes a priority. These three prevention stages are discussed later in Chapter 3.

As a field of study, ergonomics deals with many areas including the following (Fig. 1.1):

1. Study of anatomy, physiology, and psychology
2. Applied anthropometry

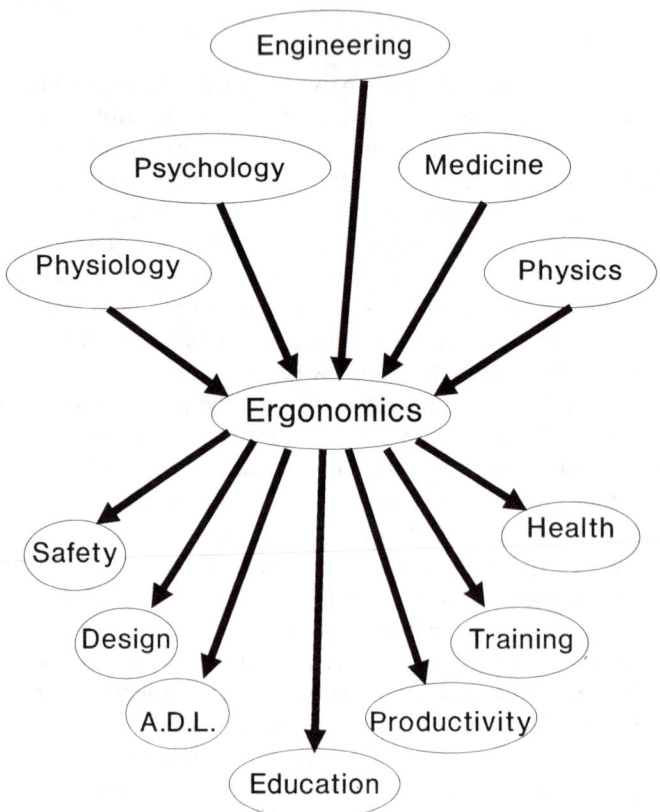

FIGURE 1.1. Ergonomics integrates knowledge of many scientific fields in order to deal with complex issues related to work, health, safety, and the well-being of humans.

3. Posture
4. Body mechanics (posture in motion)
5. Biomechanics (application of Newtonian mechanics to the human body)
6. Human cognitive processes
7. Engineering design of equipment, facilities, and environmental conditions
8. Safety (preventing actual trauma and cumulative trauma)
9. Health (environmental stressors influencing health)
10. Rehabilitation
11. Training
12. Manual handling of materials
13. Employment screening
14. Functional capacity assessment

THE BASIS OF THE ERGONOMIC APPROACH

The classical ergonomic approach to improving human performance and to the solution of health and safety problems is based on the study of human

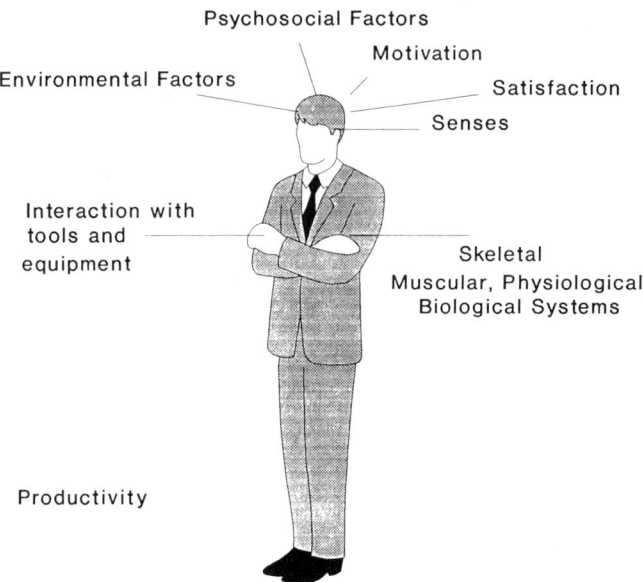

FIGURE 1.2. Human performance and productivity depends on environmental factors, psychosocial factors, work factors, and physiological factors.

4   Ergonomics in Back Pain

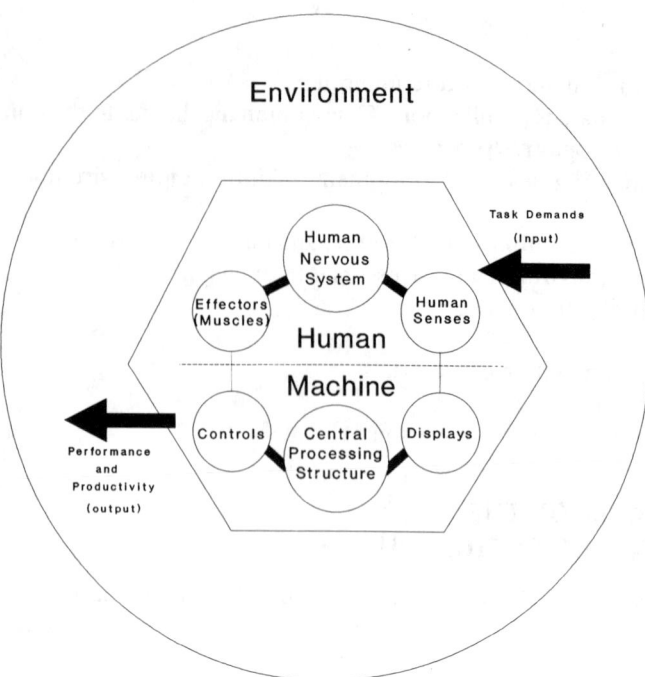

FIGURE 1.3. A model of the human-machine system showing its elements, input, output, and the environment. Environmental factors may include noise, temperature, vibration, dust, fumes, co-workers, etc.

characteristics; recognition of human capacities, abilities, and limitations; and the application of this knowledge to the analysis and design of tools, equipment, and the total environment (Fig. 1.2). Thus the application of ergonomics relies on an understanding of the interaction between people and machines (equipment, chairs, VDTs, etc.). This *human-machine system* (HMS) has three main components (Fig. 1.3).

1. **The human component** Comprised of all human characteristics: anatomical (structural), physiological (functional), and psychological (behavioral) elements
2. **The machine** Comprised of all the equipment, devices, tools, etc. with which the human being interacts (Fig. 1.4).
3. **The environment** Comprised of physical (heat, noise, vibration, etc.) and social (family, friends, job, organization, etc.) elements

In order to design an *ideal* HMS and provide a match between people and the surroundings, ergonomics recognizes four important strategies.

Ergonomics: Definition and Scope 5

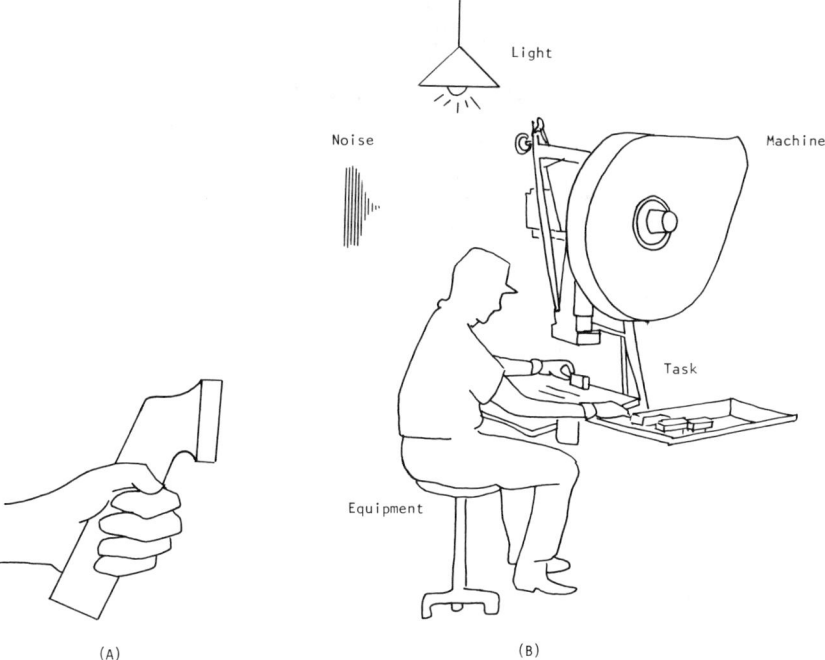

FIGURE 1.4. (A) An example of a simple human-machine system (adopted from Khalil, 1972). (B) An example of a more complex human-machine system.

1. Reduce stress Stress can be physical and/or mental (Fig. 1.5). Stresses are usually imposed by the environment in which a person exists (Tichauer, 1979). It can be imposed by a piece of equipment that is poorly designed, by being forced to assume an awkward biomechanical posture, by living or working in unhealthy environmental conditions, or by having a conflict with a co-worker or a supervisor. If the level of stress exceeds human tolerance limits, performance and productivity will decline, and safety and health will deteriorate. Stresses in the workplace and the environment should be controlled and reduced whenever possible. If stress cannot be removed, individuals should be taught ways to manage stress and deal with its sources.

2. Design Machines and equipment should be designed based on recognized human characteristics. Tasks should also be designed for ease, efficiency, and safety.

3. Match Job demands and people's abilities should be matched. It is necessary to recognize and identify the problems inherent in an HMS and thereby make recommendations for design of a better system. When there is

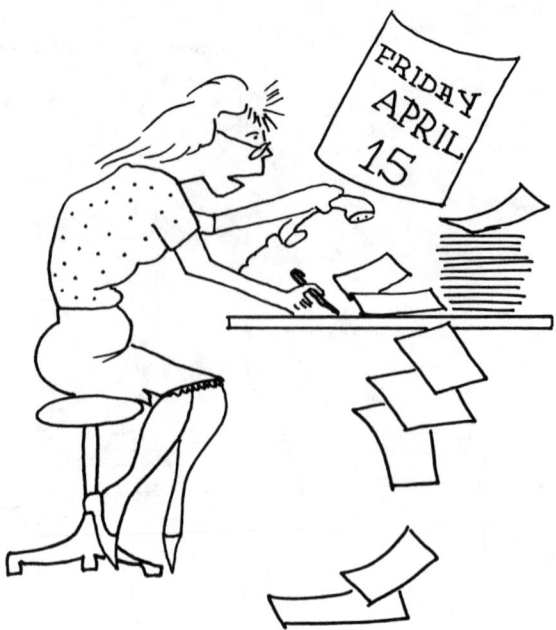

FIGURE 1.5. Stress in the workplace and in daily life can be caused by many factors. It is a major source of human suffering and may lead to musculoskeletal strain.

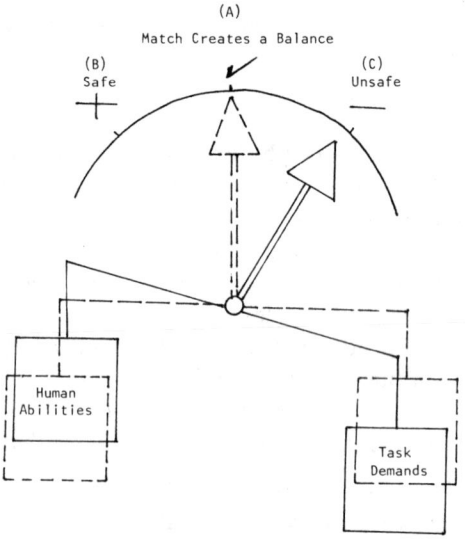

FIGURE 1.6. Ergonomics seeks optimal match between people and their work/task/environment in order to ensure a safe, productive lifestyle. (A) Task demands match human abilities—optimal environment (safe and efficient). (B) Human abilities exceed task demands—safer human-machine system. (C) Task demands exceed human capacities—injury is more likely to happen.

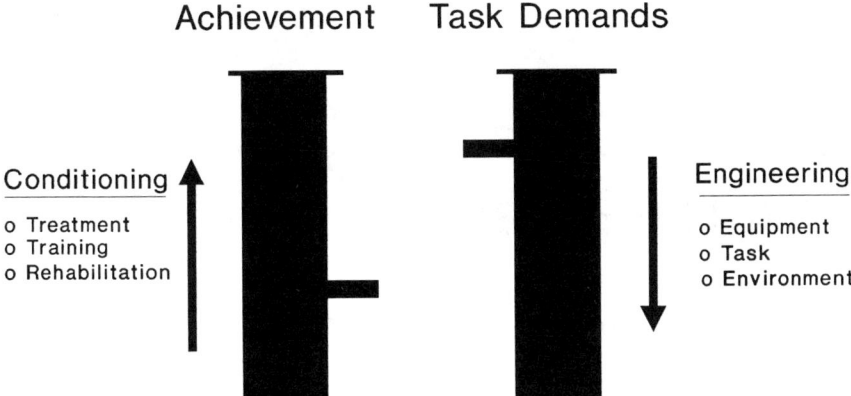

FIGURE 1.7. Human abilities can be measured on an achievement scale. These abilities can then be compared to the demands of the task. If *achievement* is less than *task demands*, human abilites should be increased (through training, rehabilitation, etc.), otherwise, task demands should be reduced (through engineering measures) in order to match human abilities.

a mismatch between the human abilities (physical and behavioral) and job demands, then the result can be performance decline, injury, health problems, and potential disability and suffering (Fig. 1.6, 1.7).

4. Educate and train People should be educated to improve their knowledge and awareness of their environment and trained to increase their tolerances to the stress of the environment (for example, exercise to improve endurance to physical stress).

This classical ergonomics approach contributes significantly to health and safety in the primary prevention of injury or illness. The same approach can be extended to include secondary prevention (rehabilitation) and tertiary prevention (post-rehabilitation). The remainder of this book is devoted to discussions of these issues as they relate to low back pain in particular and musculoskeletal problems in general.

2
Low Back Pain

THE PAIN SENSATION

Pain is the primary cause of suffering and disability and is the reason most people seek medical care (Cypress, 1983). Yet pain, and the neurophysiological-psychological mechanism that produces it, continues to baffle scientists and physicians (Rosomoff, 1991). While there are over 100 subdefinitions for the word pain, pain is subjective (Fig. 2.1). It is the patient who makes the diagnosis! Pain is whatever the patient says is occurring, wherever he says it does (McCaffrey, 1980). Differences in pain, its perception, and its characteristics must be recognized in order to treat pain properly.

The nervous system is a communication network. Nerves transmit electrical impulses to the brain. When these impulses are of a noxious nature indicative of distress the result is pain. In pain medicine, pain is recognized as a sensation that arises from tissue injury or strain. The onset of pain is the result of a primary signal, which arises most frequently from the stimulation of a pain terminal, and infrequently of an axon. The pain terminals are known to be sensitive to pressure, temperature, and certain chemical algesic substances. Important to the transmission of pain is the induction of the state of hyperalgesia and sensitization of nerve fibers, particularly those associated with tissue injury. The injury need not be gross; microscopic tissue damage will suffice. Only 15% of pain fibers reach the somatic cortex or thalamus through the primary projection pathways for pain; 85% go to the visceral and behavioral brain (Mehler, 1966). In the acute phase the visceral component predominates, but the brain accommodates quickly and the behavioral brain is then bombarded continuously. Over time, a behavioral response must ensue, usually consisting of anxiety, depression, or a combination thereof. However one chooses to define it, identify it, or describe it, unresolved pain

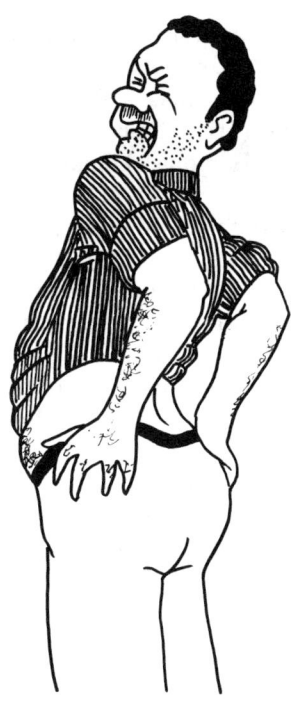

FIGURE 2.1. Low back pain strikes males and females of all ages, professions, education levels, and social status.

can lead to disability and social isolation (Holzman and Turk, 1986; Leavitt et al., 1982; Novak, 1981).

More information describing the physiological/biochemical reaction to injury and the induction of pain signals can be found in Rosomoff and Rosomoff (1991).

PREVALENCE OF LOW BACK PAIN

Low back pain (LBP) is one of modern human being's most common and complex ailments. It has been estimated that almost eight out of every ten people, at some time in their lives, will experience back pain. On any given day, over 6.5 million are in bed in the United States because of back pain, and new cases of back pain appear at the rate of approximately 1.5 million per month (Keim, 1981; Melton, 1983). Nordby (1981) estimated the number of Americans chronically disabled from LBP to be 8 million. In 1987, 34 million people in the United States suffered chronic LBP (*U.S. News & World Report*, 1987).

Other studies reported that the lifetime prevalence of LBP ranges from 60 to 90%, and the annual incidence is 5% (Frymoyer et al., 1983; Svensson and Andersson, 1983; Biering-Sorensen, 1984). Annual estimates of new cases of LBP have ranged from 10% to 15% of the U.S. population (Deyo and Tsui-Wu, 1987; Steinberg, 1982; Stanton-Hicks and Boas, 1982). Low back pain is characterized by high recurrence rate (Fig. 2.2): 60 to 80% (Dehlin et al., 1976; Hirsch et al., 1969; Rowe, 1983; Bergquist-Ulman and Larsson, 1977; Biering-Sorensen, 1984).

Low back pain is not a disease, rather it is a number of pathologic conditions, all of which cause pain (Stanton-Hicks and Boas, 1982). Backaches can strike almost anyone: the young and the old; male and female; people of all classes, races, educational levels, and professions. Low back pain ranks first among all health problems in frequency of occurrence (Bonica, 1980; Rosomoff, 1985b). It is second only to common respiratory infection as a source of lost time payment claims (Schaepe, 1982). Low back pain is the leading cause of activity limitation among young people (Kelsey et al., 1979). In the United States back pain is a leading symptom that prompts visits to physicians, second only to cold symptoms (Cypress, 1983). Low back pain constitutes the major ailment seen by chiropractors. Among the estimated 75 to 120 million annual visits to chiropractors in the United States, at least 50% are made because of low back symptoms (Brunarski, 1984).

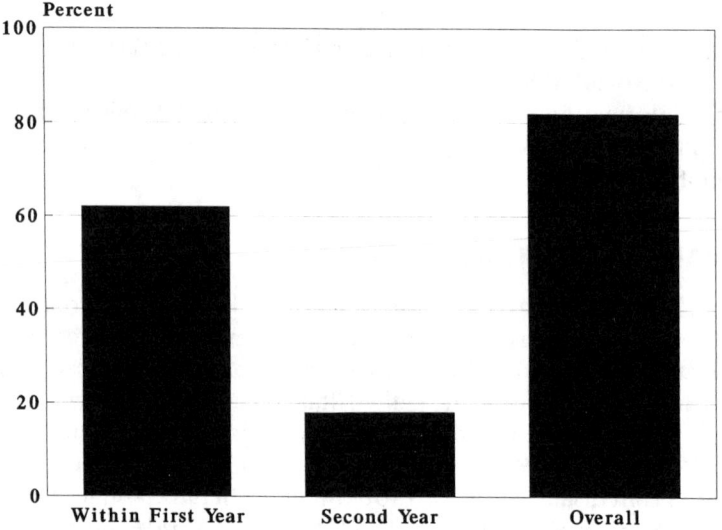

FIGURE 2.2. Low back pain is characterized by a high rate of recurrence, especially within the first year following onset.

Impairment of the back is the most common cause of chronic limitation of activity in people under age 45 and ranks third after cardiovascular disease and arthritis in those aged 45–64 (National Center for Health Statistics, 1985). Impairments of the back and spine are the major cause of disability in people between 18 and 44 years old and the third leading cause of disability in those 45 to 64 years of age (Haber, 1971). In 1974 impairment of the back and spine was the leading cause of limitation of activity and severe disability (VHS, 1974) and continues to be the leading problem today.

As indicated by the statistics cited above, the magnitude of the back pain problem has been expressed in many forms by researchers, government agencies, and health care professionals. All reported statistics convey the existence of a huge health problem that must be dealt with effectively and promptly.

LOW BACK PAIN IN THE WORKPLACE

In 1987 more than five hundred thousand back and trunk injuries occurred in the workplace (*Business & Health*, 1990) (Fig. 2.3). In the United States 1 to 2% of all employees have job-related back problems each year (Bond, 1970; Weisel et al., 1985b). Among the U.S. industrial population 28% will experience disabling low back pain at some time during their lives, while recent

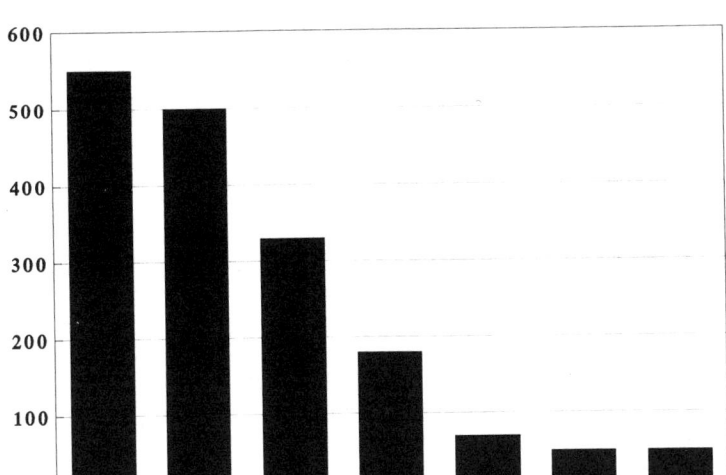

FIGURE 2.3. Injuries to the trunk happen more often than injuries to other parts of the body.

estimates suggest that 8% of the entire working population will be disabled in any given year (Oort et al., 1990). The LBP injury rate ranges from 5 injuries per one thousand workers per year in light industry to 200 injuries per one thousand workers per year in heavy industry (Schaepe, 1982). For the entire U.S. work force, estimates range from 170 to 240 million lost work days per year as a result of back impairment (Bonica, 1980). The impact of LBP is expected to increase as longevity and the average age of the work force increase (Bonica, 1980). Waddel (1987) estimates the rate of return to work for an injured individual who has been out of work for more than six months to be 50%; of those who stayed out for one year, only 25% returned to work; and those who were out for more than two years had a zero percent return to work.

COST OF THE LOW BACK PAIN PROBLEM

Low back pain is often associated with functional disability, economic and social consequences, and enormous burdensome effects on the individual sufferer, industry, the health care system, and society. Low back pain is the most expensive health care problem in the 30–50 age group. In most industries LBP is the top item in compensation payments. Its cost—on the basis of lost earnings, worker compensation and disability payments, and expenses for medical care—exceeds that of any other single health disorder (Rosomoff, 1985b) (Fig. 2.4). Although low back injury accounts for only one out of every five compensable injuries, it demands 33% of all compensable needs: $4.6 billion annually (Oort et al., 1990). Approximately 74.2% of workers with reported LBP, return to work within one month. More than 7.4% of workers with spinal disorders, however, stay out for more than six months; these cases are responsible for

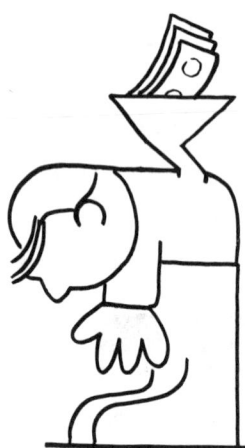

FIGURE 2.4. The sinkhole: low back pain places an enormous burden on the economy and consumes billions of dollars annually.

75.6% of the overall compensation and medical costs attributable to low back injuries (Oort et al., 1990). Other researchers (Frymoyer et al., 1983) reported that after three months only 5% of patients have persisting symptoms of LBP, yet this population accounts for 85% of the costs in terms of compensation and lost work due to LBP. Snook (1983) showed that 25% of back injury cases account for 90% of the cost (Fig 2.5).

Low back pain accounts for 40% of all lost work days. Industry spends $7 billion a year on sick leave (Carbines and Schwartz, 1987). In 1978 alone an estimated $14 billion was spent for the treatment of LBP in the United States (Schaepe, 1982). More recent estimates suggest that medical spending to alleviate back pain totals about $24 billion a year (*Fortune*, 1992). Each back injury is estimated to cost an average of $19,000 (Carbines and Schwartz, 1987). Approximately 240 million work days/year are lost because of back disorders in the United States (Bonica, 1980). Also, nearly 30% of all compensation claims are LBP claims (Schaepe, 1982). Carbine and Schwartz (1987) estimate that chronic pain accounts for an estimated $70 billion a year in medical costs, lost work days, and compensation payments. The percentage attributed to LBP alone was not given.

The number of back surgeries was estimated to be between 200,000 and 450,000 (Nordby, 1981). Nordby estimates that actual medical-related expenses for each back surgery has been placed at $18,000 per patient. Associated losses, such as lost benefits and interrupted income, were estimated to be $22,000. These figures are undoubtedly higher in today's prices. Based on the 1981 figures, and assuming indirect cost of injury to be four times the direct cost (Heinrich, 1959), the following scenario in estimating cost is plausible:

Number of operative procedures	200,000 to 450,000
Average cost per case ($18,000 + $22,000)	$40,000
Total direct cost	$8 to $18 billion
Indirect cost (4 × direct cost)	$32 to $72 billion

This puts the total cost associated with back problems in the United States at $40 billion, and potentially reaching $90 billion annually.

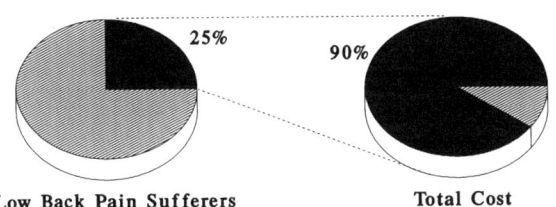

FIGURE 2.5. The less than 25% of LBP sufferers who do not improve spontaneously consume approximately 90% of the total health care resources and associated costs.

STRUCTURE OF THE BACK

In order to understand the potential origin(s) of low back pain, it is necessary to know the structure and function of the human body and in particular this critical region of the body—the back.

The Skeletal System

The skeletal system is the framework of the human body, which houses the internal softer structures such as the brain, heart, lungs, and viscera. It also provides attachment points of the muscles. The skeleton consists of some 200 separate bones attached together by means of ligaments. The skeleton may be divided into two distinct parts: the axial skeleton (Fig. 2.6), which is composed of the skull, the vertebral column, and the ribs; and the appendicular skeleton, which is composed of the pectoral and pelvic girdles and the bones of the appendages. The axial skeleton is more rigid and protects the soft structures, while the appendicular skeleton (Fig. 2.7) is highly flexible and movable. Bone movement is achieved through the action of muscles and is based on the principles of levers. Skeletal or voluntary muscles are the ones that provide such movement. The structure and function of the skeletal and muscular systems determine the method and capability of human movement and strength.

Vertebral Column

The vertebral column is the main central support structure of the body. It is the container of the superhighway of nerves controlling various body functions. It consists of 33 vertebrae (Fig. 2.8). The articulation between the column and the head and between the individual vertebrae is such that movement is allowed in many planes, but structural strength is maintained.

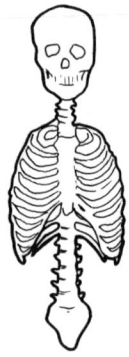

FIGURE 2.6. The axial skeleton.

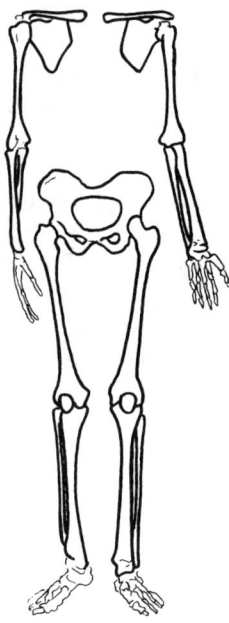

FIGURE 2.7. The appendicular skeleton.

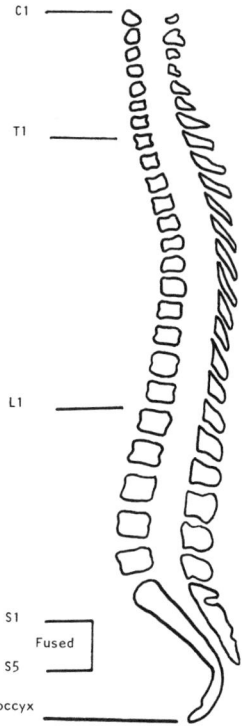

FIGURE 2.8. A sagittal section of the spine showing its configuration.

The vertebrae are supported by cartilage that acts as a cushion between each two vertebrae. Normally the vertebrae are divided into five groups: cervical, thoracic, lumbar, sacral, and coccygeal as follows:

1. There are seven cervical vertebrae making up the neck portion of the column (Fig. 2.9). The first and second cervical vertebrae are called the atlas and axis, respectively, and are the points of articulation that account for the magnificent mechanical mobility of the head. Motion takes place between the skull and the atlas. Flexion and extension, for example, occur between the skull and the atlas. Rotation of the head is accomplished as a result of motion between the atlas and axis. The atlas is firmly attached to the skull and in rotation moves as one with it.

2. There are 12 thoracic vertebrae, distinguished from all others by the facets they contain to allow articulation with the ribs (Fig. 2.10).

3. Five lumbar vertebrae compose the lower part of the back (Fig. 2.11). These are the largest vertebrae, as any engineer might easily expect, in order to support the heavy load of the upper part of the body (approximately 60% of the total body weight). These are distinguished from the thoracic vertebrae by the absence of rib facets.

4. The five sacral vertebrae are fused in the normal adult to form the triangular sacrum.

5. The number of coccygeal vertebrae may be as low as three or as high as five. Normally these are fused to form the taillike coccyx, a small triangular bone occupying a position below the sacrum.

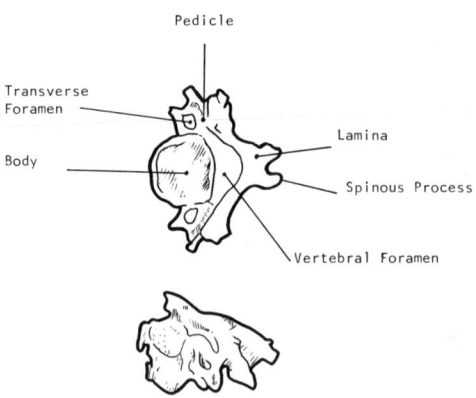

FIGURE 2.9. A front and top view showing the structure and components of a cervical vertebra.

Low Back Pain   17

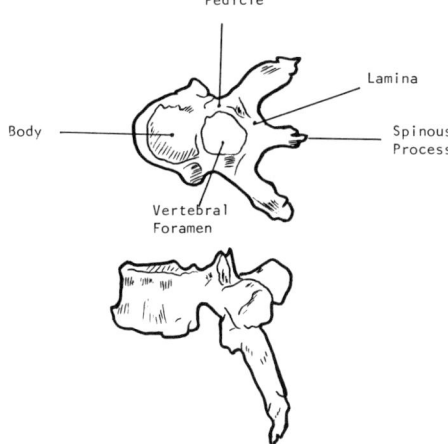

FIGURE 2.10. A front and top view showing the structure and components of a thoracic vertebra.

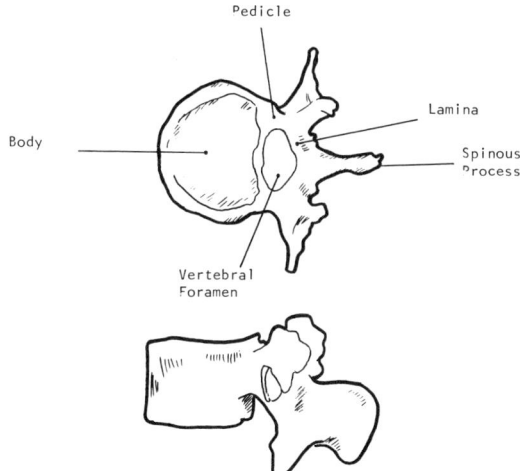

FIGURE 2.11. A front and top view showing the structure and components of a lumbar vertebra.

The lumbosacral angle (LSA) shown in Fig. 2.12 is important in determining the shape of the spinal column. It also is important in determining the components of forces acting on the fifth lumbar first sacral disk space and the surrounding hard and soft tissue structures (Fig. 2.13). For human beings with *normal* posture the LSA is approximately 41°.

18   Ergonomics in Back Pain

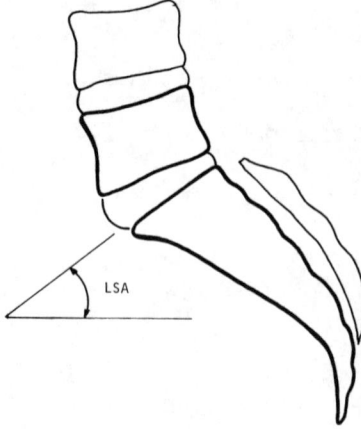

FIGURE 2.12. The lumbosacral angle (LSA) is approximatley 41 degrees when the subject is standing erect.

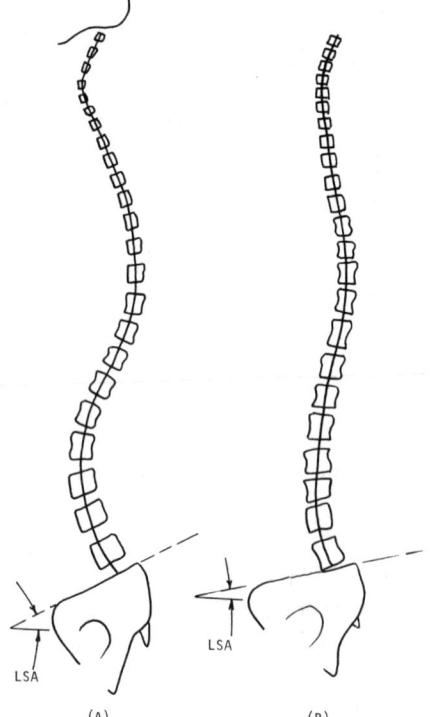

FIGURE 2.13. The effect of changing the sacral angle on the shape of the spinal column. Decreased angle from A to B changes the shape of the spinal column and flattens the pelvic and L5/S1 support structure.

The Central Nervous System, Spinal Cord, and the Nerves

The entire human body is controlled by the nervous system. The central nervous system consists of the brain and spinal cord. The spinal cord runs through the foramena of the vertebrae. The peripheral nervous system consists of all the motor and sensory nerves connecting between the spinal cord (Fig. 2.14) and the periphery of the body (muscles, skin, senses, etc.).

The Muscular System

Muscles provide the motive power necessary for movement of body parts. There are three types of muscles in the human body: sketetal muscles (also called voluntary or striated), smooth muscles, and the unique cardiac muscle. Skeletal muscles connect to bones and provide support and movement of the skeletal system. Muscles connect to bones by means of tendons. Each muscle has an origin and an insertion. These are the points of attachment of the muscle to the bones. The origin is the more fixed end of the attachment of a muscle to a fixed bone, and the insertion is the place of attachment of the muscle to the bone that moves. Most movements require coordination of a group of muscles. A muscle can act as a prime mover (agonist) or in opposition of a prime mover (antagonist). Prime movers supply the main power of movement contraction, while the antagonists provide control through degrees of relaxation. Fixators control movements at proximal points, so the prime movers can act on the distal points. This reduces undesired and unnecessary movement. Synergists cooperate with other muscles (for example, to aid the agonist for smooth movement).

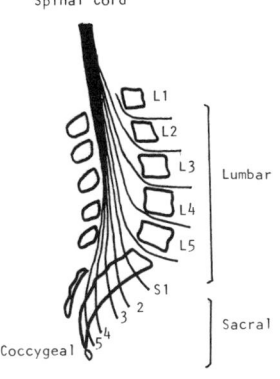

FIGURE 2.14. The spinal cord and the relation of nerve roots to the lumbosacral spinal levels.

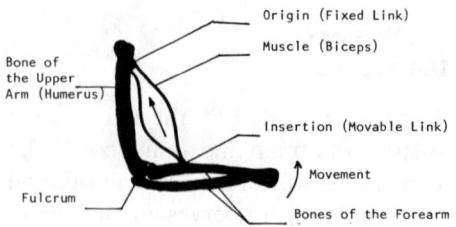

FIGURE 2.15. Origin, insertion and action of a skeletal muscle.

Muscles of the Trunk The trunk is supported in its posture by a number of muscles. Major back and hip muscles are presented in Table 2.1 with their anatomical description. Fig. 2.16 through Fig. 2.20 illustrate the relative location of a number of these muscles and their action.

TABLE 2.1   Muscles of the Trunk

Muscles	Action	Origin	Insertion
Quadratus lumborum	Lateral flexion rotation, extension of trunk	Iliac crest	Last rib and transverse processes of upper lumbar on vertebrae
Sacrospinalis	Extends trunk	Sacrum and adjacent iliac crest and lumbar/thoracic vertebrae	Ribs, spines, and transverse processes
Latissimus dorsi	Aids in adduction, extension, and inward rotation of arm	Six lower thoracic vertebrae, lumbar vertebrae, iliac crest, and outer surface of lower four ribs	Upper portion of humerus
Ilio-psoas	Flexes femur	Lumbar vertebrae and iliac fossa	Lesser trochanter of femur
Gluteus maximus	Extends femur and rotates it outward	Coccyx, iliac crest, sacrum and coccyx	Upper end of the femur
Gluteus medius	Abducts femur and stabilizes hip	Outer surface of ilium	Lateral surface of greater trochanter
Adductor brevis, longus, magnus	Adducts femur	Pubis and ischium	Linea aspersa of femur
Trapezius	Adducts scapula	Occipital protuberance down to the last thoracic vertebrae	Lateral one-third of clavicle and spine of scapula
Serratus anterior	Abducts scapula	Upper nine ribs	Vertebral border of scapula

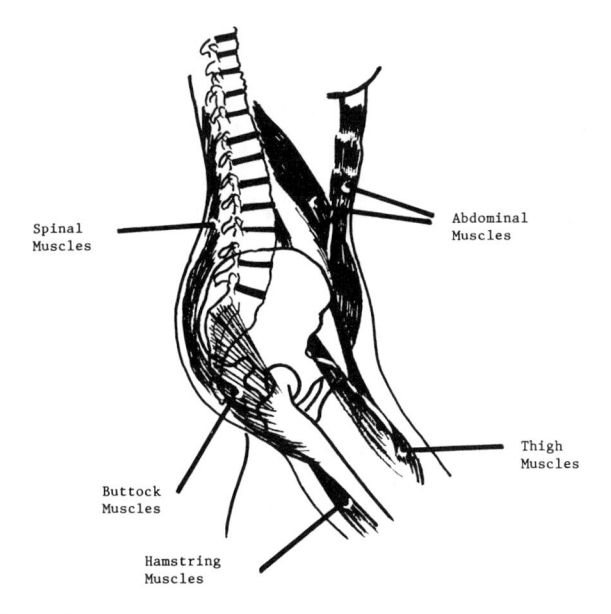

FIGURE 2.16. The major muscles providing spinal support. These are also involved in the mechanics of spine-hip mobility.

The Spine

The spine, or back, is therefore a loosely articulated group of bones that can be converted into a rigid lever arm by contraction of the paraspinal muscles. The lower extremity complete the functional unit by the movement of their muscles. The back and hips form a complex system of hard and soft tissue that works in unison to maintain posture or affect movement. Therefore, in discussing low back pain, one needs to appreciate the role of the hips, which

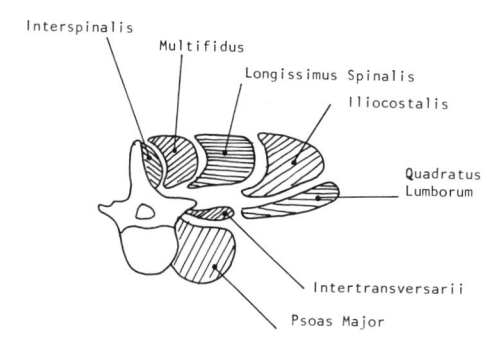

FIGURE 2.17. Muscles of the trunk shown in a unilateral transverse plane cross section.

22 Ergonomics in Back Pain

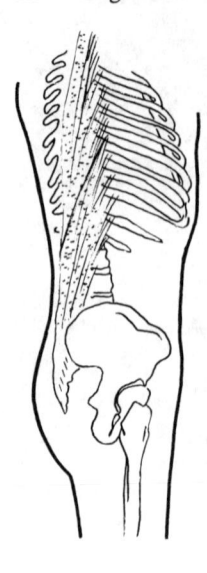

FIGURE 2.18. The sacrospinalis (erector spinae) act to extend the trunk and maintain erect posture. The fibers originate on the lower, posterior part of the sacrum and adjacent rear part of the iliac crest and lumbar/thoracic vertebrae. The insertion on the ribs, spinous, and transverse process of the thoracic and cervical vertebrae.

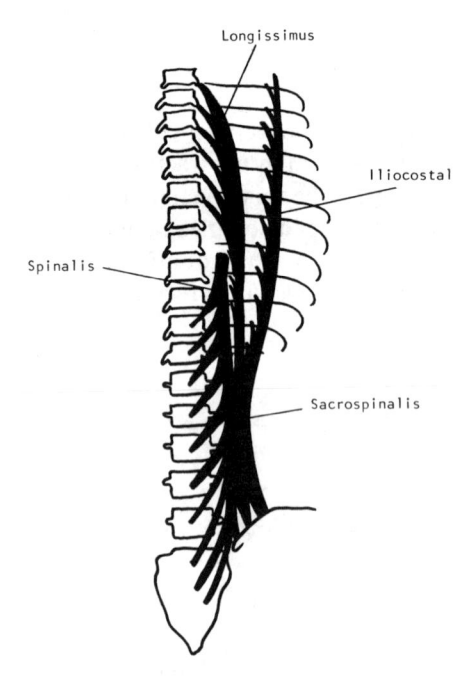

FIGURE 2.19. The extensor muscles of the spine, showing the many points of origin and insertion.

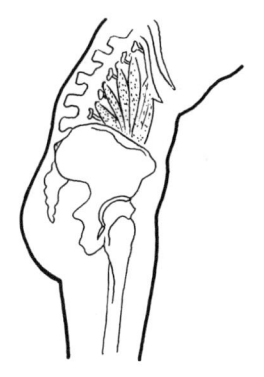

FIGURE 2.20. The quadratus lumborum muscle flexes the trunk. It originates on the rear part of the iliac crest and inserts on the lower border of the 12th rib and on the transverse processes of the upper 4 lumbar vertebrae.

control back and leg movement and which can, when mechanically insulted, produce back and lower extremity pain.

ORIGINS OF LOW BACK PAIN

Many physicians and researchers do not consider low back pain a disease, rather it is one or more pathologic conditions that can trigger pain (Stanton-Hicks and Boas, 1982). Conventionally, the causes of LBP are grouped under four categories (Table 2.2).

1. Muscular/Ligamentous
2. Structural
3. Discogenic/Neurological
4. Other disorders

TABLE 2.2   Potential Origins of Low Back Pain

1. **Muscular/Ligamentous**
   - *Tension*: resulting from stress and nervous tension.
   - *Trauma*: acute injury or cumulative type.
   - *Strain*: small tears within the muscle/tendon, either acute or chronic. Acute comes as a result of sudden stress, chronic is usually the result of repeated stress.
   - *Sprain*: injury to the ligaments that hold bone to bone.
   - *Postural imbalance*: creates uneven stresses on the musculoskeletal system.
   - *Spasm/Contracture*: muscle contraction that produces restricted ranges of motion; a chemical phenomenon wherein the traumatized muscle produces an uncontrolled contraction, with pain, tenderness, vasoconstriction, decreased blood supply, and an energy deficit contracture (Fig. 2.23).
   - *Weakness*: poor muscle tone.
   - *Myofascitis*: inflammation and tenderness of the muscle and the sheaths that envelop the muscle known as the fascia.

2. **Structural**
   - *Spondylolysis*: a defect of the bony segment joining the articulations above and below a given segment, mainly thought to be congenital, infrequently post-traumatic hyperextension.

TABLE 2.2 *(Continued)*

- *Spondylosis*: degenerative changes in all aspects of the disk. A condition in which the disk is absorbed as a result of mechanical stress causing the spinal segment to collapse, bones to deform and spur, and the vertebra to displace.
- *Spondylolisthesis*: a condition of forward displacement of the body of one vertebra on the vertebra below it, commonly occurring at the L5-S1 level when congenital or at L4-5 when degenerative (Fig. 2.24).
- *Facet dysfunction*: (also known as sublux facet joint or facet syndrome): a partial dislocation of the spinal joints.
- *Osteoporosis*: loss of bone content (Fig. 2.25).
- *Scoliosis*: abnormal curvature of the spine (Fig. 2.26).
- *Compression fractures*: usually affects the bodies of the vertebrae. They are the result of bone weakening with loss of bone content (Fig. 2.27).
- *Dislocation*
- *Degenerative disease*
- *Osteoarthritis*: a degenerative disorder that affects the facet joints and disk, causing general breakdown of the cartilage of the joint and bony growths, or spurs, around the edge of the joint.
- *Annular tears*
- *Spinal stenosis*: narrowing of the spinal canal. A degenerative disease caused by spondylosis in the intervertebral disk and osteoarthritis of the facet joints. Bony spurs form around the facet joints of the spine, causing them to encroach posteriorly into the spinal canal. The enlarged joints narrow the canal, prevent the nerves from exiting, and in some cases cause nerve root entrapment syndrome (Fig. 2.28).
- *Tumors*: abnormal growths in the body involving vertebrae (osteoid-osteoma, Paget's disease), also pelvic and bone tumors (multiple myeloma).
- *Trauma*: application of load exceeding the strength of the tissue.
- *Spina bifida occulta*: a condition of incomplete closure of the posterior bony elements of the vertebrae at the lower spine (Fig. 2.29).

3. **Discogenic / Neurological**
   - *Disk herniation*: Also known as rupturing, slipping, or bulging. Herniation of the nucleus pulposus through the fibers of the annulus fibrosus. Mostly occurring in younger people (30 and 40 years). Most common at L4-5 and L5-S1 levels.
   - *Nerve irritation*
   - *Tumors*: involving nerve roots or meninges (neurinoma or meningioma)

4. **Others**
   - *Infectious disorders:* bacterial infection through the rich blood supply in the vertebral body disk space (for example, tuberculosis or osteomylitis—a serious bone infection).
   - *Metabolic disorders*: due to nutrient deficiencies (for example, osteoporosis).
   - *Congenital disorders*: not necessarily genetic or hereditary. Among these is the transitional vertebrae: four lumbar vertebrae (a condition called sacralization) or six lumbar vertebrae (condition called lumbarization).
   - *Circulatory disorders*: hardening of the arteries (arteriosclerosis), causing obstruction of the blood vessels going down the leg; also, vascular insufficiency such as varicose veins.
   - *Inflammatory disorders*: most common is rheumatoid arthritis.
   - *Psychoneurotic problems*: stress, hysteria, anxiety, hypochondriasis, malingering.
   - *Toxicity*: poisoning due to pollutants, industrial waste, radiation, lead, etc. May lead to cancers and/or nerve irritation.

Low Back Pain 25

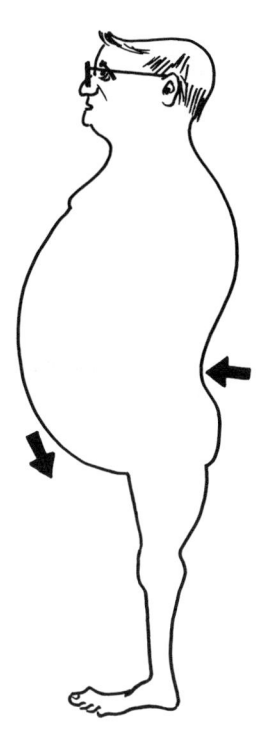

FIGURE 2.21. Poor posture due to obesity places great demands on the spine and may lead to back pain.

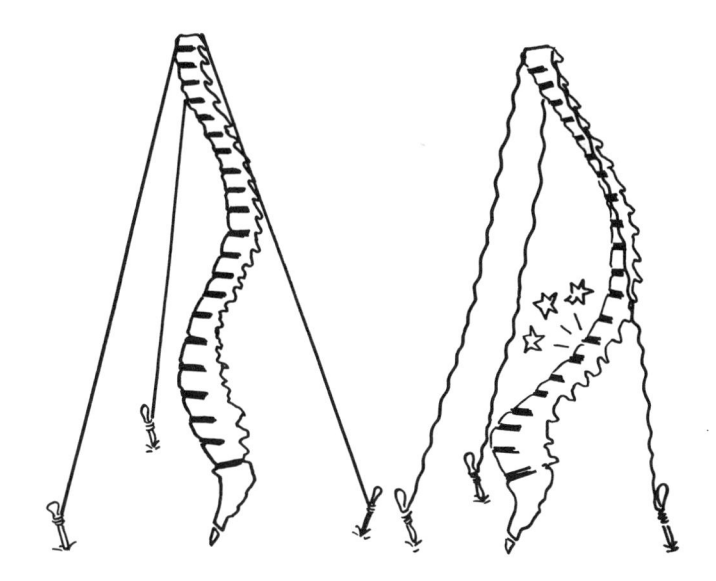

FIGURE 2.22. The paravertebral muscle provide critical support to the spinal column. Muscle weakness causes biomechanical imbalance of the column.

26   Ergonomics in Back Pain

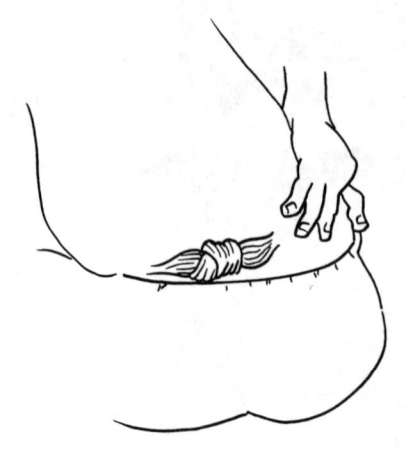

FIGURE 2.23.   Sudden movements, muscular overload, and many other factors can cause the back muscles to contract and remain in a state of spasm leading to low back pain.

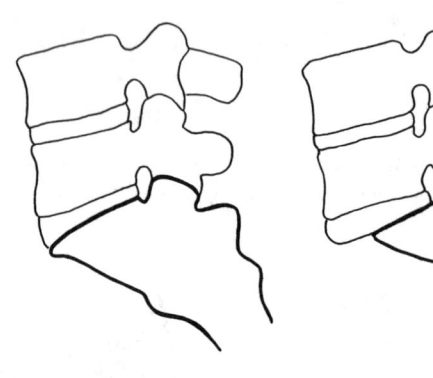

FIGURE 2.24.   Spondylolisthesis.

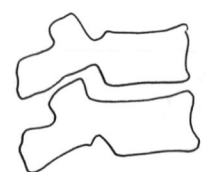

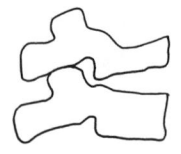

FIGURE 2.25.   The effect of osteoporosis on vertebral configuration.

Low Back Pain 27

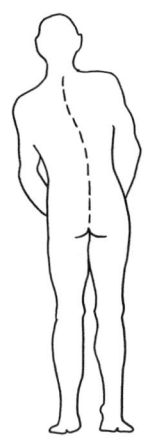

FIGURE 2.26. Scoliosis.

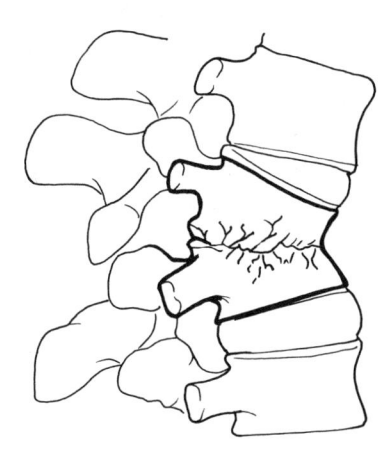

FIGURE 2.27. Compression fracture.

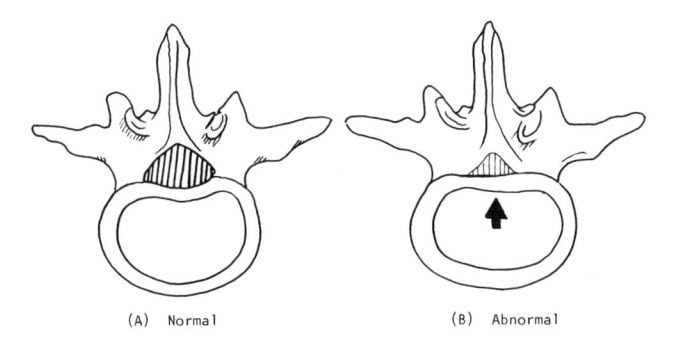

(A) Normal   (B) Abnormal

FIGURE 2.28. Spinal stenosis decreases the effective space for spinal nerves.

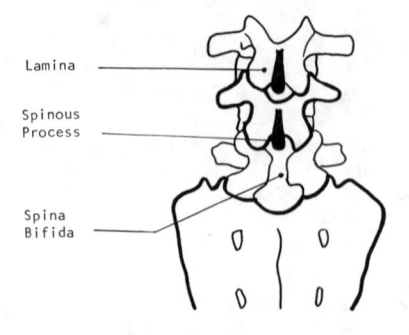

FIGURE 2.29. At L5, there is absence of a portion of the lamina and spinaous process (spinal bifida.)

RISK FACTORS

Many risk factors associated with the onset of low back pain have been identified (Table 2.3). They vary widely based on the population studied and the conditions under which the study was conducted. The main risk factors are summarized in Table 2.3. Whether these factors represent the cause of injury, events leading to injury, or results of the disability is unclear (Frymoyer, 1988). Specifically, in the workplace LBP is often associated with industrial-type activities, such as driving heavy equipment and lifting. Available statistics have shown that people who are involved in sedentary-type and other nonindustrial activities, such as nurses, are equally prone to suffer low back pain (Khalil, Asfour, Moty et al., 1985). In a sample of 265 patient

TABLE 2.3 Risk Factors

1. Physical Factors		
Posture	Strength	Flexibility
Body build	Reflexes	Aerobic capacity
2. Individual Factors		
Age	Weight	Previous injury
Nutrition	Fitness level	Education
Income	Alcoholic use	Medical history
Degeneration	Smoking	
Gender	Height	
3. Psychological Factors		
Depression	Marital discord	Family problems
Anxiety	Job dissatisfaction	Personality traits
Attitudes toward work		
4. Environmental Factors		
Prolonged sitting	Years on job	Climate
Accidents	Driving	Lifting (amount of weight,
Vibration	Slips and falls	frequency, twisting)

with LBP, the authors classified their job activities according to the *Dictionary of Occupational Titles* (US *Department of Labor*, 1987). It was found that while 34% of the patients were involved in some kind of heavy work (such as construction workers and heavy equipment operators), 36% of them performed light-type work (such as sedentary occupations) (Fig. 2.30). It is becoming increasingly evident that job activities are not the major cause of low back pain. The most important and detrimental factor in the onset of back pain appears to be related to the way in which work activities are performed. In this same sample, the most common event leading to low back pain and injury was slipping and falling (41.5%), followed, as a distant second, by injuries due to lifting and carrying (24.9%) (Fig. 2.31–2.33).

PROFILE OF THE BACK PAIN PATIENT

Individuals with chronic pain are either characterized by or having one or more of the following conditions or both:

- Prominent complaints of pain
- Physically impaired
- Behavioral changes
- Changes in lifestyle
- Helpless and hopeless
- Weak
- Assumes the sick role
- Feel inadequate

Job Demand Classification* of Workers with Chronic LBP

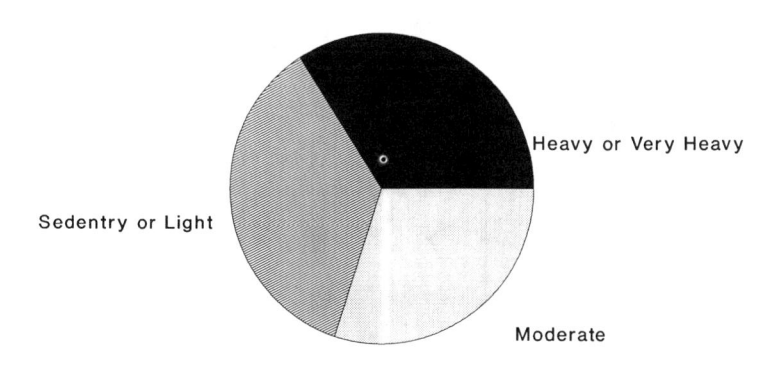

* Classification according to DOT.

FIGURE 2.30. In a study of the pattern of employment among workers suffering from chronic low back pain, those involved in heavy-type jobs were found to be equally likely to sustain a back injury as compared to those in sedentary or light-type jobs (job classifications are according to the Dictionary of Occupation Titles, DOT).

30   Ergonomics in Back Pain

Causes of Injury in Workers with Chronic LBP

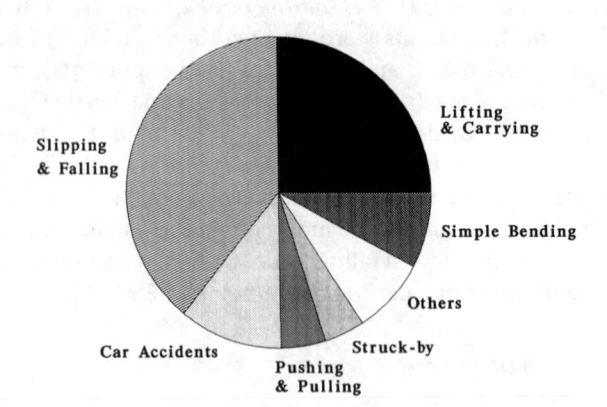

FIGURE 2.31.   Our findings have shown that slips and falls are the greatest cause of chronic low back injury followed by lifting and carrying as a distant second.

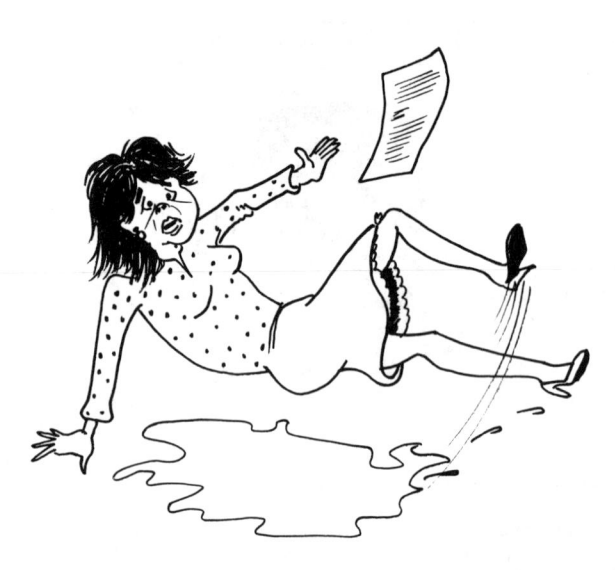

FIGURE 2.32.   Slipping and falling on wet surfaces is an unexpected, uncontrolled event that led to low back pain and injury in many cases.

Low Back Pain   31

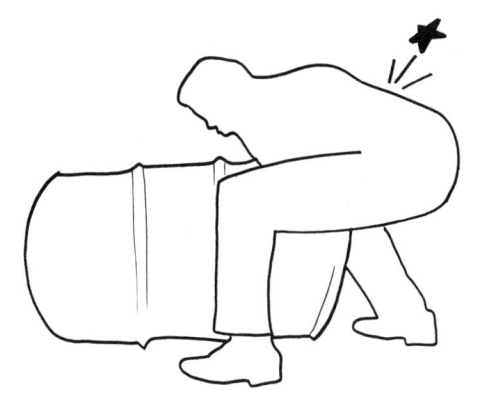

FIGURE 2.33. Improper methods of lifting and handling objects place significant amounts of stress on the lower back and may result in injury. There are many human, task, and engineering variables that affect the method of lifting.

- Socially dependent
- Emotional depression
- Drug dependent
- Alcohol dependent
- Seek hospitalization
- Played the invalid role
- Unable to cope
- Physically dysfunctional
- Poor work history
- Psychologically disturbed
- Dependent
- Psychiatrically disturbed
- Sexual problems
- Fearful
- Family and home problems
- Litigation
- Low self-esteem
- Unable to deal with stress
- Poorly motivated
- Dissatisfied with their job
- Problems with role reversal
- Angry
- Resentful
- Lonely
- Hostile
- Angry with insurance
- Withdrawn

Contributors to this profile of the low back pain patient are the family, the medical community, the attorney, the rehabilitation specialist, the insurance company, and the employer (Rosomoff, 1985b). Hadler (1978) suggests that chronic low back pain can be thought of as a medical predicament that is compounded by health care providers or the social system.

ACUTE VERSUS CHRONIC PAIN

Pain is a very complex subjective experience that is very difficult to describe in objective terms. From a therapeutic point of view, pain can be classified broadly as acute and chronic.

Acute pain represents the body's reaction to a biological or physical injury, distress, trauma, infection, inflammation, surgery, or illness. Acute pain is identified at onset.

The term *chronic pain* is used to describe a multifaceted subjective pain, in addition to a host of behavioral, socioeconomic, and/or psychosocial complaints, all usually accompanied by disproportionate physical findings. Pain is chronic when it continues long after the original trauma condition has resolved. In contrast to the phenomenon of acute pain, the concept of chronic pain has emerged as pain that persists past the normal time of healing (Bonica, 1953). In reality, this time period may be less than one month, but more commonly thought to be more than six months (Rosomoff and Rosomoff, 1991). Three months has been proposed as the point of division by the Subcommittee on Taxonomy of the International Association for the Study of Pain (Merskey, 1986). This definition of chronic pain is an arbitrary designation, which unfairly views pain as a chronological event rather than a physiologic function. A better definition of chronic pain has been offered recently: A continuum of noxious input, like that of acute pain, but modulated and compounded by the prolonged or recurrent nature of the chronic state, and further complicated by a multitude of economic and psychological factors (Rosomoff and Rosomoff, 1991).

THE CYCLES OF PAIN

The chronic pain patient usually gets entrapped into three closed-loop cycles (Fig. 2.34). The first cycle can be called the *physical deconditioning cycle*. The patient tries to compensate for his/her pain by adopting unnatural and restricted postures. This, in turn, results in muscle spasms; reduced ranges of motion in joints; shortening or contractures of muscles, ligaments, and tendons; and a maladaptive gait. These adaptations lead to increased pain, part of which could be in structures not originally involved. The second cycle is called the *drug cycle*. The patient attempts to relieve the pain by taking drugs. With time, the body develops tolerance to the drugs, and additional dosages are needed to suppress the pain. Some even amplify the perception of pain, and none is fully effective. The third cycle is the *depression and anxiety cycle*. Because of pain and reduced functional capabilities, the patient becomes depressed and anxious. This, in turn, leads the patient to focus more on the pain.

DISABILITY, IMPAIRMENT, AND DYSFUNCTION OF LOW BACK PAIN PATIENTS

To treat a patient with chronic pain condition these three cycles must be broken:

Low Back Pain   33

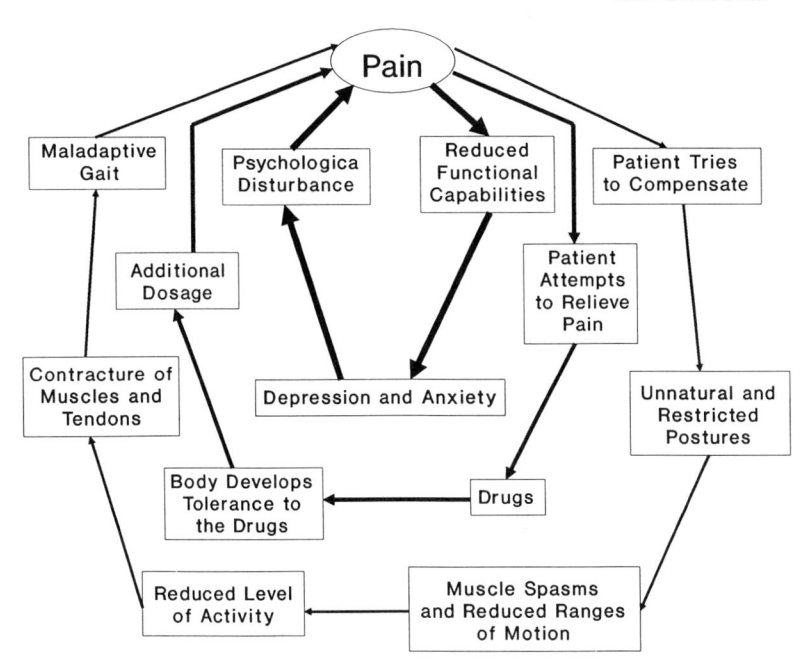

FIGURE 2.34. The three pain cycles. From inside outwards: the depression/anxiety cycle, the drug cycle, and the physical deconditioning cycle.

1. Disability
2. Impairment, and
3. Disfunction.

Disability and impairment are two terms that are being used interchangeably, and mistakenly. An impaired individual may not necessarily be disabled. *Disability* is a limitation in performance. It is determined based on ability/inability to perform activities of daily living (occupational and/or nonoccupational). Disability could be partial or total. Disability can be described in terms of residual functional capacity in relation to task demands and can be determined through the use of a variety of assessment instruments (medical, vocational, physical, psychological, and others).

Impairment describes anatomic or functional abnormality or loss: natural or induced reduction in one or more of a body organ's function. At the present time, the American Medical Association Guidelines remain one of the most useful instruments to rate impairment for medico-legal purposes. Other impairment rating systems have been adopted by some states. An impaired individual does not necessarily have to be disabled. The former applies to human body characteristics, while the latter relates to

34   Ergonomics in Back Pain

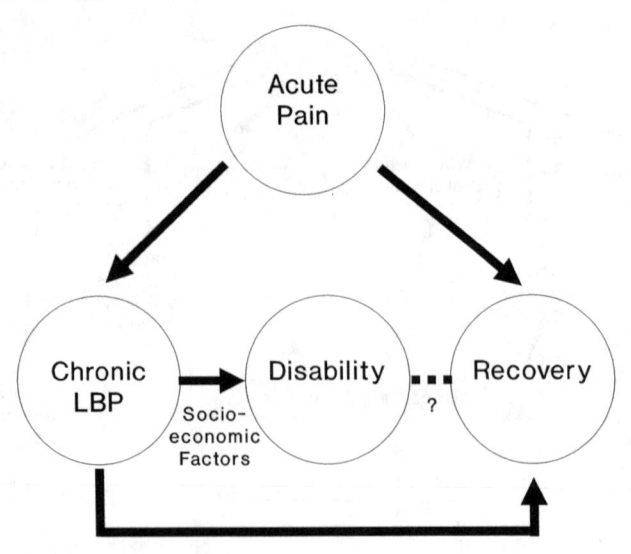

FIGURE 2.35. The house of disability: an individual may recover from an acute injury or a chronic condition. Disability is the product of chronicity in the prescence of other factors.

performance of a job function or demands of daily living. Pain is not rated as an impairment unless it is substantiated by objective medical findings (Brena and Turk, 1988). However, according to the World Health Organization's definition of pain, chronic pain can be viewed as a sensory impairment affecting the neuromusculoskeletal system (Brena and Turk, 1988).

Low back pain in itself does not create disability. It can be thought of as a medical predicament (Hadler, 1978). It is only when a multitude of socio-economic factors enter into the equation that chronic pain and disability occur (Fig. 2.35).

Impairment and dysfunction are also sometimes misunderstood. Most LBP patients have a dysfunction that can be treated, and they may not be impaired at all.

Chronic Back Pain	+	Work loss
(Dysfunction)	+	Hospitalization
	+	Compensation
	+	Inability to lead normal life
	=	Disability

3
Low Back Pain Management and the Role of Ergonomics

Chronic low back pain is a complex problem that cannot be managed solely by the expertise of health care professionals. It is becoming increasingly recognized that the problem of chronic LBP requires a multidisciplinary approach that addresses patients' problems holistically: physically, behaviorally, socially, as well as occupationally. This requires professionals from each of these fields to interact in a simultaneous effort to prevent or control the problem at its various stages (Table 3.1).

Ideally, the problem of LBP should be controlled prior to its occurrence. This process is referred to as *primary prevention*, where emphasis should be on designing a safer human-machine system (matching workers to work and designing safe environments). Even though efforts are being made to achieve this goal, low back injuries continue to occur at an alarming rate. Once injury takes place, the priority becomes to control and prevent disability and minimize the time out of work. This can be achieved through effective comprehensive rehabilitation, with the goal of preparing the individual to return to a productive lifestyle within a safe environment. This process is called *secondary prevention* or disability prevention. Despite the efforts at

TABLE 3.1 The Three Stages of Injury Prevention: Primary, Secondary, and Tertiary

Injury Condition	Prevention Stage	Objective
1 Pre-Injury	Primary	Prevention of Injury
2 Post-Injury	Secondary	Prevention of Disability
3 Post Rehab.	Tertiary	Prevention of Reinjury

ERGONOMIC CONTRIBUTIONS TO LOW BACK PAIN

Pre-Injury	Post-Injury	Post-Rehabilitation
o Pre-employment Screening	o Evaluation	o Follow-up
o Job Placement	o Education	o Task Modification
o Training	o Treatment	o Job Modification
o Workplace Design	o Job Simulation	o Workplace Modification
o Task Design	o Job Modification	o Environmental Modifications
o Job / Task Modification	o Work Conditioning	o Training
o Environmental Modification		
o Education		

FIGURE 3.1. A summary of ergonomic contributions at the three stages of injury prevention.

achieving maximum medical and physical improvement, recurrence of injury or pain remains a disturbing phenomenon. The natural step in this process is to design effective programs to prevent reinjury. Prevention of reinjury is referred to as *tertiary prevention*, where emphasis should be on ensuring that the rehabilitated individual continues to a) maintain functional capacities and b) perform safely in work and leisure time activities in a well-engineered environment.

Therefore, it is evident that good engineering, awareness, and physical fitness are three common factors in all of these stages. Ergonomics deals with all of these issues, and its applications have proved to be effective in addressing the problem from all perspectives. A major advantage is that ergonomic contributions to the solution of the LBP problem can take place in all three stages (Fig. 3.1). The role of ergonomics in each of the three stages is discussed in the following sections. Examples of ergonomic interventions are presented in chapters 4 through 10.

ERGONOMICS IN THE PRE-INJURY STAGE

The thrust of the ergonomic approach is to eliminate unsafe situations that can contribute to injury, rather than just take corrective actions after a mishap. In this prevention stage (also known as primary prevention or line of first defense) the implementation of ergonomic guidelines and principles for the reduction of musculoskeletal stresses and accidents is the best approach to avoid injury and reduce the individual's exposure to risk factors. It has been demonstrated that low back injuries can be reduced by 30% when ergonomic approaches for the reduction of undue effort and work stresses are implemented (Snook et al., 1978). In the pre-injury stage, good design of tasks and work or home environments are essential. Equally important is that workers' awareness of the environment and their knowledge of ergonomics and the biomechanical principles for the design of the workplace and task performance should be increased. Workers should be trained to know their physical capabilities and limitations. Prevention and control of injuries through education and training should be individualized, with a sufficient degree of flexibility to accommodate methods of working. The concepts must be transferred to home and recreational activities, and should become an integral part of daily activities.

Proper education reduces the incidence of injuries to the lower back among industrial workers (Hall and Iceton, 1983). Through early evaluation and proper intervention at the workplace, the number of patients reporting low back symptoms can be reduced by 41% at job sites; days lost from work can be decreased by 60%; surgical operations can be decreased by 88%—resulting in a financial savings of 55% (Weisel et al., 1985b). The specific guidelines for the use of ergonomic principles in injury prevention are given in the intervention strategies in chapters 4, 5, and 7.

THE POST-INJURY REHABILITATION STAGE

Once low back pain develops, it usually comes under the supervision of the health care professionals. The line of defense against disability becomes the secondary prevention strategy.

The Role of the Medical Community

The medical approach to the management of low back pain problems relies heavily on traditional treatment modalities of the injured individual. The evaluation and management of the LBP problem varies widely among the different health care providers. Typically a clinical evaluation is performed followed by a prescribed treatment approach.

Clinical Evaluations
Comprehensive evaluation of low back pain patients is largely interdisciplinary. Most rehabilitation programs usually are composed of one or more of the following clinical evaluations: physician evaluation, physical therapy evaluation, occupational therapy assessment, psychological examination, and vocational evaluation.

Physician's Evaluation
The objective of the physician's evaluation is to examine the neurologic and orthopedic aspects of the human body to provide a diagnosis of the ailment. Physicians rely on medical history, patients' self-reports of pain level and loca-

tion, medication intake, and functional deficiencies. They may make use of such procedures as X-rays, CT scans, electrodiagnostic studies, myelograms, discograms, thermograms, and other laboratory studies. In addition to conventional anatomic and pathologic data, these evaluations emphasize aspects such as documentation of the mechanism and the precise location of the pain at the onset of injury; the patient's general appearance, gait pattern, posture, muscle strength, flexibility; and soft tissue factors (tenderness, spasms, swelling, trigger points, etc.). Table 3.2 summarizes a physician evaluation profile.

Physical Therapy Evaluation

This type of evaluation emphasizes the different aspects of the soft tissues and the musculoskeletal system, such as muscle strength, ranges of motion, gait, spasms, swelling, pain pattern, etc. The methods used in this category are usually manual; for example, the evaluation of muscle strength is done manually and is often reported on a scale from 0 (no strength) to 5 (normal strength). While yielding numerical data, this measure involves some degree of subjective input on the part of the therapist and usually lacks sensitivity to adequately describe patient's function or progress. The reliability of these measures is also questionable—in evaluating strength, for example, the assessment is done manually and the outcome could very well depend on the

TABLE 3.2 Profile of Physician Evaluation

1. **History**
2. **Physical exam**
   a. Observation
   b. Palpation
   c. Testing
   - spasms
   - mobility
   - tenderness
   - toe-heel standing
   - straight leg raising
   - muscle strength testing
   - skin dermatomes
   - head compression
   - distraction test
   - flexibility of spine and hip
   - deformity
   - neurologic deficit signs
   - posture
   - squatting
   - stretch test
   - symmetry
   - atrophy
   - Lasegue's test
   - motor/sensory tests
   - leg length and circumferences
3. **Diagnostic tests**
   - radiographs
   - computer-assisted tomography [CT scan]
   - magnetic resonance imaging [MRI]
   - thermography
   - electrodiagnostic tests
   - myelography
   - blood tests
   - bone scans
   - discography

physical strength of the evaluator and the time of evaluation. Recently, new technology has enabled the introduction of testing equipment (such as electronic goniometers and muscle testing machines) that permit quantitative measurement of human functions. Therapists are encouraged to utilize this new technology in their evaluations and documentation.

Occupational Therapy Evaluation
Occupational therapy evaluation serves to describe how a patient functions in activities of daily living. The evaluation includes activities such as bed activities, self-care activities, social activities, leisure activities, walking, standing, sitting, climbing stairs or ladders, traveling, driving, carrying and lifting, pushing and pulling, and other vocational and avocational activities. This type of evaluation provides descriptive information about the degree of independence, tolerances, endurance, speed, and attitude of the patient while performing these activities.

Psychological Evaluation
This examination reveals a great deal about the patient's mental state, behaviors, coping styles, and the effects of pain or injury on his/her personality. There are various types of psychological tests. Most of these are designed to elicit responses that can be translated into numerical values and compared with the performance of other people.

Vocational Evaluation
This evaluation has many objectives. Some of these are (1) to gather impressions and facts about the patient's self-reported vocational abilities, difficulties, interests, goals, and work personality; (2) to assist the patient to achieve educational and vocational goals that are feasible; and (3) to help set up the initial steps toward the vocational goals by having the patient participate in activities and simulations designed to help overcome problems of adjustment. Vocational evaluation is performed through interviews and vocational tests and are reported in the form of scores.

Summary
Existing clinical evaluation methodologies often produce qualitative and subjective descriptions of the patient's function. Collectively they provide an insight on the patient's function at the time of evaluation. More attention to the establishment of quantitative measures of patients' functional abilities would greatly enhance the effectiveness of these evaluations. The development and implementation of objective, quantitative scientific methodologies for the evaluation of function fall under the realm of ergonomic science.

Medical Treatment and Management
The Basis of Medical Intervention

The following discussion is relevant to the two most common diagnoses rendered for low back pain: namely, (1) nerve root compression from a herniated disk and/or degenerative bony changes, and (2) myofascial pain syndrome. This discussion is intended to present two commonly accepted theories that may explain the mechanism of LBP.

Herniated Disk The symptom of back pain extending into the leg, commonly known as sciatica, is traditionally presumed to be due to *pinching* or compression of one or more spinal nerve roots. When degenerative changes occur in the disk, the nucleus pulposus (NP) tends to squeeze out, usually through the weakest area of the annulus (Fig. 3.2 and Fig. 3.3). This may produce compression or irritation of nerve roots of the spinal canal. Disk herniation is fundamentally a release of the nuclear material from the confinement of the enveloping annulus fibrosus capsule (Mixter and Barr, 1934). Herniation of the nuclear material may result from excessive forces, repeated stresses, prolonged tension, or the presence of faulty annulus.

The traditional treatment of disk herniation has been the surgical removal in laminectomy. Currently, this practice is severely challenged. A large percentage of adults with no back pain symptoms show some form of disk herniation when an X-ray of the spine is taken. About 0.8% of Swedish adults and 0.2% of American adults have had herniated disk operations (Frymoyer et al., 1983). Surgical procedures fail to relieve pain at all in 30% of patients, and after five years only 10% of these operations have provided satisfactory relief (Trief, 1983). An estimated 25% of the laminectomies done each year (30% for disk removal and spinal fusion) are failures (Kornfeld, 1982).

It should be noted that disk degeneration occurs naturally in humans. The frequency and degree of disk degeneration is directly related to age. By the end of the fourth decade, 40% of the population shows signs of degenerative disk disease (Hult, 1954). In Hult's sample the frequency of degeneration is higher, but not statistically significant, in individuals who had an episode of

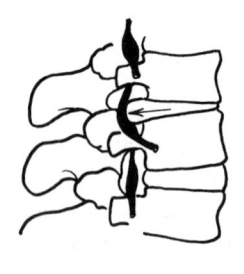

FIGURE 3.2. The theory of disk herniation: the nucleus pulposes outflows.

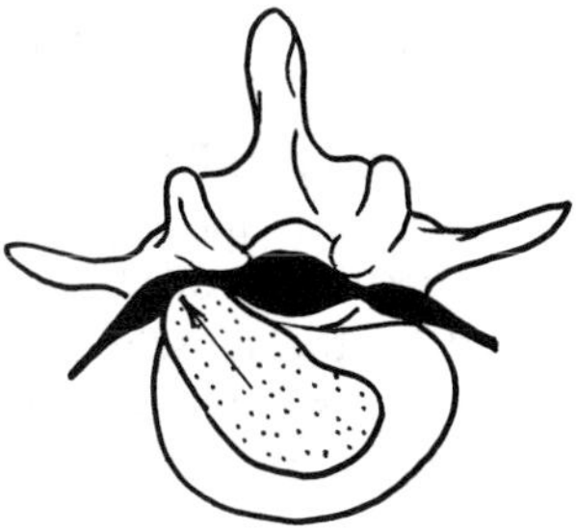

FIGURE 3.3. Disk herniation is thought to result in the outlfow of the nucleus pulposes, thus impinging on the nerve root.

back pain. By the time individuals reach the sixth decade of life, the disks are usually dried out, with minimal chances for herniation.

Do herniated disks produce pain? After more than 50 years of allegiance to the Mixter-Barr concept of the ruptured disk (Mixter and Barr, 1934), continuing failure to solve the dilemmas of LBP makes it time to reconsider and look elsewhere to other sources of pain. Physiological studies demonstrate that, except for transient pain when first impacted, sustained nerve root compression does not produce pain (Wall, 1974). There may be numbness or loss of function—for example, when one's leg falls asleep—but it should not be a painful event. Sufficiently sustained severe nerve root compression can produce nerve root dysfunction in the form of sensory, motor, or reflex loss, but deficits are not present in the majority of patients. Therefore, other causes must be considered as the agents giving rise to pain (Rosomoff, 1985a). It follows that successful definition of the origin of pain, with appropriate treatment, could result in relief or prevention of pain and disability, without resorting to surgery with its attendant risks of failures.

Myofascial Pain Syndrome There is a strong belief that the most frequent cause of low back pain is tear and inflammation of the soft tissue including ligaments and fascia. The medical diagnosis of such pain is given as myofascial pain syndrome (MPS). Simons and Travell (1983) and the International Association for the Study of Pain Subcommittee on Taxonomy (IASP, 1986) discuss the physiologic and pathologic mechanisms underlying the syndrome of myofascial pain. Myofascial pain syndrome is widely diagnosed and has been classified either as a diffuse or specific syndrome. Diffuse MPS has been defined as diffuse aching musculoskeletal pain associated with multiple discrete predictable tender points and stiffness. Myofascial trigger points are self-sustained, hyperirritable foci located in skeletal muscle or its associated fascia, which produce referred pain, decreased range of motion, decreased muscle strength, and tender muscles. Specific MPS may occur in any voluntary muscle with referred pain, local and referred tenderness, and a tense shortened muscle. The pain has the same qualities as that of diffuse syndromes. Diagnosis depends on demonstration of a trigger or tender points and reproduction of the pain. A trigger point is a point in the body that produces pain when pressed.

The neurophysiological support for this thesis can be found in Rosomoff (1985a) (Fig. 3.4). From inspection of human anatomy, it is inescapably clear that low back injuries have associated soft tissue abnormalities because the protective covering and support offered by the muscle represents the bulk of the anatomy affected. Even if the forces applied reach sufficient strength to herniate or rupture an intervertebral disk, these forces must be transmitted first through the overlying soft tissue (annulus fibrosus, ligaments, tendons, and muscles) that binds the spine together as a functional unit and maintains its integrity and stability. These tissues, when injured, undergo a breakdown of the cell membranes and biosynthesis of chemicals. This induces a state of hyperalgesia, which is followed by a pain signal that evolves when excessive mechanical stimulation occurs or when chemical compounds are produced as a reaction to the injury (Vane, 1983). The nerve root itself does not originate the pain signal. Nociceptors are stimulated to originate the transmission of the signal.

The thesis here is that the disordered musculoskeletal system is responsi-

```
Forces Exceeding Structural Tolerance Limits
                    ↓
              Tissue Injury
                    ↓
             Archidonic Acid
                    ↓
        Biosynthesis of Chemicals
                    ↓
   State of Hyperalgesia, Vascular Instability,
     Inflammatory Reaction and Contraction
                    ↓
              ( Pain Signal )
```

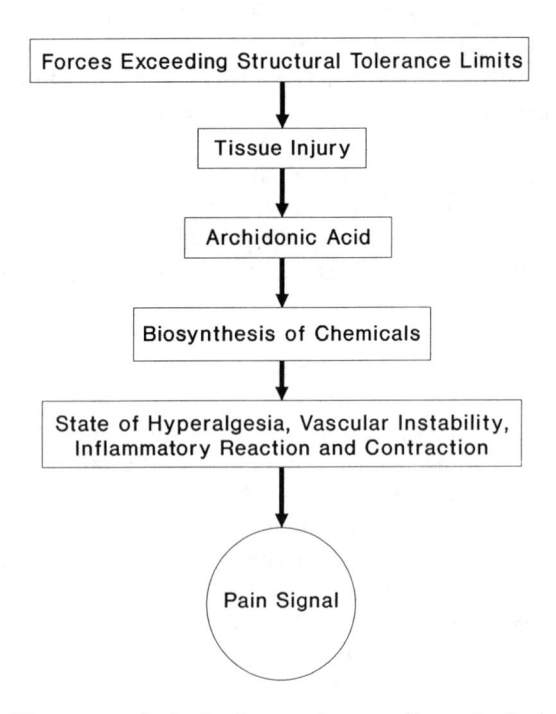

FIGURE 3.4. The process of pain signal generation according to the thesis of myofascial syndrome.

ble for initiating these phenomena. These structures are extraspinal in the surrounding paraspinal muscles, buttocks, hips, and legs. These peripheral sites and syndromes are treatable. When treatment is successful, function is restored and pain is alleviated without the need to correct any number of intraspinal pathological entities that have traditionally been designated as one of the causes of pain and neurologic deficit.

Whether the site of injury is a disk, or hard tissue, a soft tissue component is always, present. The neurophysiologic evidence presented earlier demonstrates that nerve root compression, per se, as the cause of LBP is not a tenable thesis. Soft tissue injury and the body of knowledge that supports the generic concepts of inflammation and reaction to injury are the replacement.

A number of MPSs associated with LBP have been recognized by Simons and Travell (1983). Some of these will be discussed briefly for the sake of completeness.

Types of Myofascial Pain Syndrome

1. Quadratus lumborum syndrome The typical history is of a quick, stooping movement when the torso is twisted. Pain occurs around the iliac crest, gluteal areas, tronchanter, groin, and deep in the buttock. The patient has pain with weight bearing, twisting, and stooping. No pain is associated with coughing. Night pain occurs; back movements are restricted; a pelvic tilt is present. Tenderness is found deep paraspinally, but pain is referred to the sacroiliac and buttock areas.

2. Gluteal syndrome This syndrome produces pain about the buttock, coccyx, medial sacrum, lateral iliac crest, posterior thigh, and calf, with a radiating pattern typical of sciatica. Tenderness is found at the sacrum medially and at the attachment of the gluteal muscle along the iliac crest and tronchanter. Pain is referred into the buttock, posterior thigh, and lateral leg.

3. Ilio-psoas syndrome This syndrome is often found with quadratus lumborum syndrome. Ipsilateral back pain and anterior thigh pain are found. Gait is characterized by external rotation and flexion at the hip. The ilio-psoas is contracted.

4. Rectus abdominis syndrome This syndrome produces bandlike low thoracic and low lumbar pain, but the trigger points are anteriorly placed at the origin and insertion of the muscle. Lax abdominal muscles and poor conditioning are the source of this condition.

Approaches to Low Back Pain Management

The management of the back-injured victim is far from simple (Rosomoff and Rosomoff, 1991). A low back pain treatment system must be capable of identifying and dealing with the patient's problems in a concise way. These problems can be categorized as sensory, perceptual, psychological, psychosocial, environmental, and biomechanical. An early referral to a competent medical center may prevent simple sprain from becoming a total disability and can avoid the behavioral consequences that are certain to develop if chronicity becomes established.

In general, the goals of all LBP management approaches (treatment and rehabilitation) should focus on the following (Fig. 3.5):

1. Reducing chronicity
2. Preventing disability
3. Restoring function
4. Returning the patient to a productive lifestyle

Various medical treatment approaches have been advocated by different health care providers in response to the magnitude of the LBP problem. These treatment approaches can be classified broadly under two distinct categories (Fig. 3.6).

1. Conservative (either passive, also called nonphysical, or aggressive, also called boot camp)
2. Nonconservative (surgical)

Describing the elements and comparing the efficacy of these approaches is beyond the scope of this book. However, the most commonly utilized management methods are mentioned below.

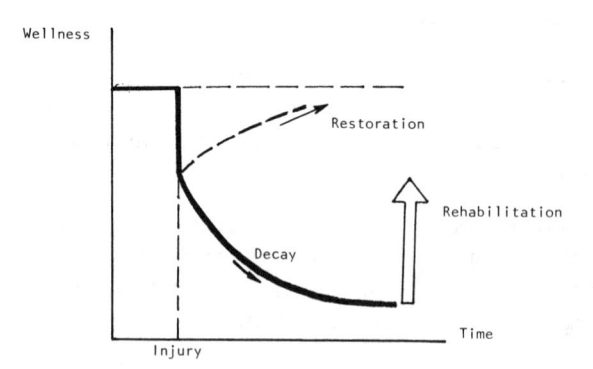

FIGURE 3.5. Injury results in a decline in human health over time. The objective of rehabilitation is, therefore, to restore human health and well-being over a relatively short period of time in order to prevent chronicity.

MANAGEMENT OF LOW BACK PAIN

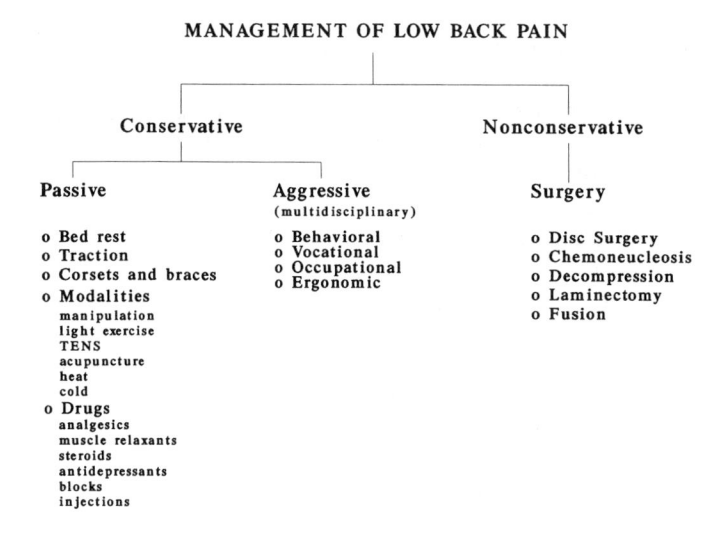

```
                    Management of Low Back Pain
                    ┌──────────────┴──────────────┐
              Conservative                  Nonconservative
         ┌────────┴────────┐                      │
      Passive         Aggressive                Surgery
                   (multidisciplinary)
  o Bed rest         o Behavioral            o Disc Surgery
  o Traction         o Vocational            o Chemoneucleosis
  o Corsets and      o Occupational          o Decompression
    braces           o Ergonomic             o Laminectomy
  o Modalities                               o Fusion
      manipulation
      light exercise
      TENS
      acupuncture
      heat
      cold
  o Drugs
      analgesics
      muscle relaxants
      steroids
      antidepressants
      blocks
      injections
```

FIGURE 3.6. Classification of the approaches to the management of low back pain and the main elements of each approach.

Bed Rest and Immobilization Rest and immobility are the immediate natural reaction of humans to injury and pain. Immobility will increase pain; cause disuse, atrophy, and weakness; slow healing; and demineralize bone, resulting in functional disability (Cailliet, 1980). Therefore, bed rest should not be indicated for chronic LBP patients.

The Aggressive (Multidisciplinary) Approach Although experts agree that traditional approaches to treating LBP have failed, they continue to disagree over the diagnosis and treatment of the problem. They do, however, agree on the basic concepts of a multidisciplinary rehabilitation approach for the patient with chronic pain (Ng, 1981). This approach constitutes the foundations for most pain centers.

Pain centers are traditionally viewed as facilities where patients are sent for the treatment of chronic pain, after conventional management has failed and no further supervised disease-oriented care is deemed appropriate (Rosomoff and Rosomoff, 1991). Multidisciplinary pain centers (MPC) approach chronic pain from a number of perspectives. These centers deal with the treatment, management, and study of the science of pain (algology). They have been classified according to one or more of the following characteristics:

1. Size (physical facility and space)
2. Personnel (medical director, program director, program coordinator, physicians, physiatrists, administrators, admissions, physical therapists, occu-

pational therapists, counselors, psychologists, ergonomists, vocational rehabilitation specialists, and nurses)
3. Program components (medical, administrative, secretarial, inpatient, outpatient, therapy, evaluation, education, consultation)
4. Research activities
5. Training and education activities
6. Therapy (physical, occupational, behavioral)
7. Evaluation routines
8. Patient follow-up conferences

A variety of pain facilities exist around the work, ranging from unimodal pain clinics to highly sophisticated multimodal centers. Four major types have been identified (Bonica, 1988).

1. Major comprehensive pain centers
2. Comprehensive pain centers
3. Syndrome-oriented pain centers
4. Modality-oriented pain centers

With the exception of syndrome-oriented pain centers, most of these centers are spine clinics. Almost every one has an 80% to 90% population of patients with cervical spine or low back problems, so perhaps they are all improperly named (Rosomoff and Rosomoff, 1991). Their treatment approaches are often biased by the nature of the medical director.

Pain programs, centers, and clinics have been formally in existence in the United States since the early 1970s (Bonica, 1980). In 1977 there were 327 pain clinics listed, and in 1987 it was estimated that there were between 1,000 and 1,200 such pain centers in the United States (Bonica, 1988). An estimated 2,000 pain clinics or pain centers exist in the United States today. However, no two are alike (Rosomoff, 1991). This sudden proliferation puts the burden on the patients to choose which facility is capable of providing the most effective treatment. This has also presented problems for pain organizations when they wrote standards for pain programs (Task Force, 1990). Pain programs should be designed to meet the needs of the targeted populations. Admission criteria should be based on the services that can be offered and the level of expertise of its team to treat the problems (Rosomoff, 1991).

Pain centers were previously described as being multidisciplinary, inpatient, or outpatient. These centers promote physical medicine, behavioral medicine, nerve stimulation, exercise, physical therapy modalities, surgeries, electric implants, pharmacology, hypnosis, and so forth. However intended, it is now clear that no one discipline or mode of treatment will suffice (Rosomoff and Rosomoff, 1991).

Aggressive treatment of LBP emphasizes activity and exercise. Activity increases endorphin levels, which becomes an endogenous source of pain control, decreasing pain and facilitating healing (Carr et al., 1981). Furthermore, *working through pain* produces the phenomenon of stress-induced analgesia. In simplistic terms, if stress (that is, pain) is applied continuously without interruption, pain transmission will cease (like an overload of an electric system that blows the circuit breaker). The patient is pain-free for a period of time, which is a golden opportunity to apply therapy that is usually pain-provoking, like muscle stretching. Coupled with exercise-induced endorphin release, treatment can be advanced, but the patient and the treating professional must overcome the natural fear of pain, which is equated with injury. When muscles are activated intensively, depression is decreased, mobility is increased, analgesic intake is decreased, drug withdrawal is eased, and a sense of well-being is induced.

Radical (Surgical) Interventions Laminectomies, discectomies, and fusions are done seven times more frequently in the United States than in any other country (Nachemson, 1981). In 1973 there were approximately 147,000 intervertebral disks excised (VHS, 1977), with an estimated 200,000 to 450,000 back operations performed annually (Pheasant, 1977). Nordby (1981) estimates that 200,000 surgical operations to the back took place in 1974, and that in 1976 there were more likely 450,000 back operations in the United States In 1977 400,000 people in the United States were hospitalized with a diagnosis of disk displacement (VHS, 1977). This figure does not include cases of spinal fusion or other types of spinal disorders. In 1983 188,000 operations were performed in the United States for herniation of lumbar disks (Rutkow, 1986).

The available literature speaks to the fact that disk surgery is not the solution for back pain in the majority of cases. The results of multiple surgeries were reported to be worse. Waddell et al. (1979) report that beginning with the third operation, most patients in their study group were worse following their surgery than prior to it. It is clear that surgical treatment of patients is not good (Stanton-Hicks and Boas, 1982). The Quebec Task Force on Spinal Disorders reports (Quebec Study, 1987) found that of 45,000 patients only 1% of cases of low back disorder involve deficits and indications for surgical intervention, of which approximately one-half result in surgery.

It is believed that surgery for a herniated disk is indicated infrequently, particularly in persons over age 50, because the aging process causes disk degeneration, resulting in resorption or hardened bony transformation (Rosomoff, 1991). Consequently, there is no disk to remove or the bony changes make removal impossible (Rosomoff and Rosomoff, 1987). Surgery done early on the well-selected patient under 50 years of age can be successful

(Hurme and Alaranta, 1987). However, this takes place in only one-half of 1% of persons with back pain (Quebec study, 1987).

ERGONOMICS IN THE POST-INJURY REHABILITATION STAGE

The Concept of Rehabilitation Through Technology

In a state of wellness an individual has certain capacities. These capacities can be described through quantitatively measured indices. Healthy people engage in activities of daily living (ADL) and in tasks as permitted by their individual capacities. These capacities can be increased by training or exercise and diminished by age or injury.

In most cases, an instantaneous reduction of capacity occurs in one or more of the components of the human system: for example, to the muscle, to the heart, or to a joint. If this is not followed by immediate treatment or repair, a gradual decay of the system may ensue secondary to the injury, pain, or disuse. The objective of treatment and/or rehabilitation is to prevent such a decay from happening. In the secondary prevention (treatment) stage quick restoration of functional abilities becomes the most effective approach from both medical and economic points of view.

Secondary prevention is done either through medical intervention or technological intervention. Medical intervention is self-explanatory. Technological intervention implies the use of prosthetic, orthotic, and/or ergonomically inspired equipment and techniques to restore performance to a state of wellness.

The combined treatment and technological interventions improve human achievement to a certain level, which can then be compared to any job demands. If there is an agreeable match, then the injured individual is capable of performing that job or any host of jobs that have demands equal to or less than the achievement level of the individual. Job demands can also be reduced by means of engineering redesign of the job environment and/or task. Ergonomics also plays a major role in this regard. These approaches of technological rehabilitation stem from the basic concepts of the human-machine system presented in Chapter 1.

The Clinical Ergonomist as a Part of the Health Care Team

Very few researchers in ergonomics have devoted their efforts to post-injury management of pain conditions. This has always been thought of as the sole domain of the medical and health care professionals. Involvement by ergonomists in injury evaluation and low back pain management programs, however, has proved to be quite successful (Khalil, Asfour, Moty, 1985). Ergonomic reasoning has become an integral part of a multidisciplinary involvement in patients' treatment. It also permits an objective, quantitative assessment of patients' functional abilities.

The goal of rehabilitation encompasses preventing disability through functional restoration and immediate return to a productive lifestyle (Fig. 3.7). Due to the complexity of the problem, it has been well recognized that chronic pain management requires a multidisciplinary approach since no one physician or therapist has the expertise or resources to manage this condition. The health care professions that are usually involved in low back pain rehabilitation include: physicians, physical therapists, occupational therapists, nurses, vocational counselors, psychologists, and psychiatrists (Fig. 3.8). One discipline that can contribute significantly to pain management is ergonomics. The study of ergonomics deals with safety, human performance analysis, work environment, and other studies of value to the rehabilitation process. Also, due to its nature as an interdisciplinary science, it can offer solutions to many problems related to injury and its prevention.

The Ergonomics Division of the University of Miami Comprehensive Pain and Rehabilitation Center (Miami Beach, Florida) is an example of where ergonomists work daily with members of a multidisciplinary rehabilitation team to solve problems in pain management and return-to-work issues. Over the past decade, the ergonomics division has integrated its activities and resources with those of the center. With the introduction of the ergonomics division in 1981, ergonomists attempted to establish open communication

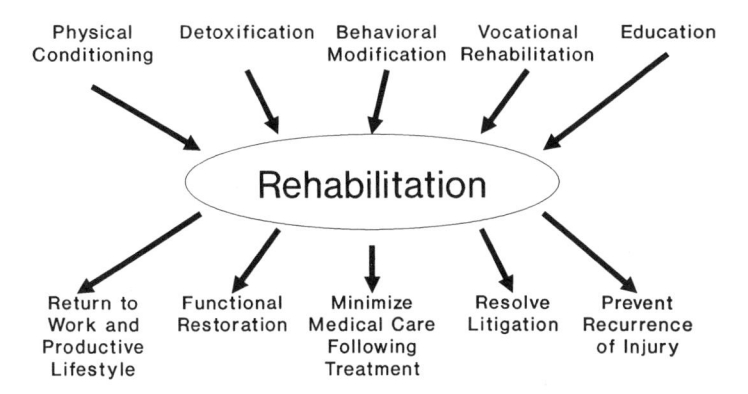

FIGURE 3.7. Goal-oriented rehabilitation programs utilize a holistic approach with input from physical, psychological, and vocational arenas in order to achieve the ultimate goal of functional restoration.

```
┌──────────────┐   ┌──────────┐   ┌──────────────┐
│ Occupational │←──│ Nursing  │←──│  Vocational  │
│   Therapy    │   │          │   │Rehabilitation│
└──────────────┘   └──────────┘   └──────────────┘
        ↕                ↓                ↑
┌──────────────┐                  ┌──────────────┐
│   Physical   │──→            ←──│   Physical   │
│   Therapy    │      Patient     │   Medicine   │
└──────────────┘                  └──────────────┘
        ↕                                ↕
┌──────────────┐                  ┌──────────────┐
│  Psychology  │──→            ←──│  Psychiatry  │
└──────────────┘                  └──────────────┘
        ↕                ↑                ↕
┌──────────────┐   ┌──────────┐   ┌──────────────┐
│ Biofeedback  │←──│Ergonomics│←──│    Muscle    │
│              │   │          │   │ Reeducation  │
└──────────────┘   └──────────┘   └──────────────┘
```

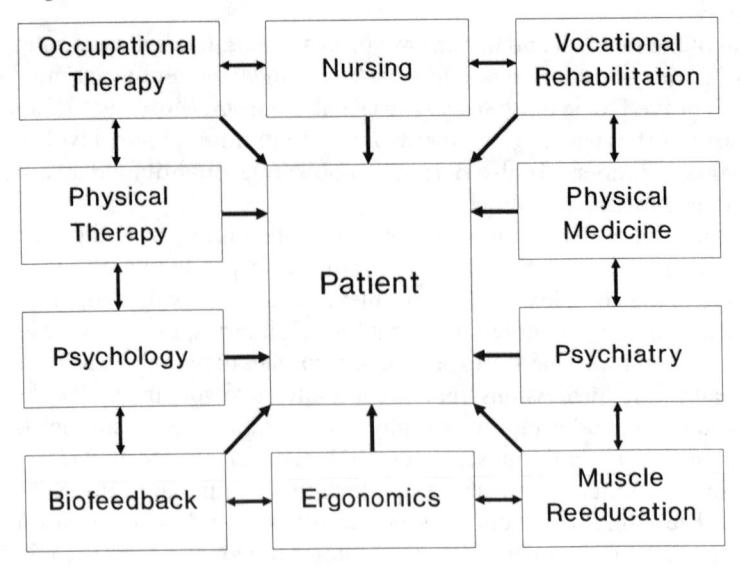

FIGURE 3.8. A model of multidisciplinary pain management: Ergonomists integrate their efforts with those of other health care professionals and work jointly for the well-being of the patient.

channels with the medical community through continuous exchange of knowledge and information pertinent to rehabilitation. It was important at that stage for example, to adopt and modify some of the principles related to human performance analysis in order to deal with injured individuals rather than healthy subjects. Initially, the health care system was skeptical about the role of *engineers* in the day-to-day care of patients. Ergonomists successfully bridged that gap and integrated their efforts with those of other disciplines (physical therapy, occupational therapy, vocational rehabilitation, Biofeedback, etc.). This has provided a unique opportunity to address many complex problems from both an engineering and a medical perspective. For the first time, this has provided the scientific basis for the rationalization of many treatment approaches. Through applied research activities, dissemination of valuable information and data was possible and new nontraditional treatment approaches and techniques were developed. It is becoming necessary to utilize this model in other rehabilitation settings especially since the introduction of advanced rehabilitation technology and disability management methods.

In the area of patient care, ergonomics contributes to the determination of the functional status of the low back pain patient through the establishment of profiles of functional abilities. This is done through a battery of quantitative measurements that help establish a human performance profile for each patient on admission and throughout rehabilitation. The goal of treatment is, then, to condition the injured individual and to restore functional levels to the *normal* capacities of healthy uninjured individuals. The performance profiles are then compared to the physical demands dictated by the job. The objective here is to determine intervention strategies for matching the physical capabilities of the individual to specific job tasks. This may require the design or modification of the workplace, tools, and/or work methods. At this stage, ergonomic job analysis, job simulation, and job-site visits are used to prepare the injured worker to reenter the productive job market and lead a normal lifestyle. Realistic job simulations are developed within the rehabilitation setting to permit patients to perform job tasks under medical supervision. The patient is taught to perform his job tasks properly, which assures him/her that he/she is capable of carrying them out. This also allows the patient and the treating physician to certify that the patient has been physically rehabilitated to handle task demands. Ergonomically established techniques and criteria are implemented in this type of activity. Designing and/or recommending appropriate seating devices, equipment, and furniture that would permit reduced work stresses is an example of such approaches. The objective is to implement ergonomic knowledge pertaining to workplace design and to make use of computer-aided technology to help patients adjust their workplace. This is done in order to minimize potential stresses due to poorly designed and/or improperly adjusted workplaces. Ergonomists also assist in the selection of jobs that match the measured functional capabilities of rehabilitated persons. This approach presents an ideal strategy for prevention of further injury. Yet another significant contribution to treatment is the development of techniques for the restoration of functional abilities through improved performance of the musculoskeletal system. Examples in this regard are techniques of muscle reeducation, strength and endurance training, and functional electrical stimulation. The development of patient education programs based on proper body mechanics, as rationalized by biomechanical models and ergonomic concepts, is essential to the comprehensive rehabilitation process. The goal is to develop and test proper techniques and methods of performing work tasks and activities of daily living for patients with back injury.

In the area of applied clinical research, ergonomics evaluates the effectiveness of treatment regimens on the restoration of functional abilities and on the reduction of pain, thus providing objective rationalization of treatment. Research is also performed to develop and evaluate devices useful in diagnosis and treatment of low back pain. Quantitative methods based on recognized approaches are used to assist the medical professionals in identifying the usefulness of tools and equipment often prescribed for use in pain management. Another significant activity is the development of prediction models of patients' daily achievements and goals throughout rehabilitation. These models are based on initial levels and vocational/avocational goals.

The contribution of ergonomics to CLBP management has proved to be quite valuable based on our experience over the past decade. At the Comprehensive Pain and Rehabilitation Center ergonomists interact with patients as well as other members of the health care team to restore function to the CLBP patient. The involvement of ergonomics in patient care and rehabilitation research should be an integral part of pain management settings. The capacity to utilize ergonomics in a clinical setting extends beyond treatment to optimization of the treatment and prognosis of low back pain.

ERGONOMICS IN THE POST-REHABILITATION STAGE

In this stage the emphasis of ergonomics is on reengineering the task and/or the environment in order to permit a more compatible and safer relationship between people with low back pain and their working or living environment.

The post-rehabilitation stage can be thought of as the third stage in a 3 stage comprehensive disability prevention cycle. In this cycle, the individual who sustains an injury experiences pain and potential disability before entering the medical system for rehabilitation. After rehabilitation several scenarios may be observed in which the individual is

- not pain-free and remains in the pain/disability cycle,
- not pain-free and returns to work (same or different job), or
- pain-free and returns to work (same or different job).

Effective acute or chronic low back pain treatment/rehabilitation approaches can succeed in achieving the goal of functional restoration and return to work. However, if no effort is made to assure that functional gains are maintained following discharge from treatment, recurrence of pain or disability may result. During the post-rehabilitation stage ergonomics contributes in the following ways:

1. Designing effective programs for continued health following hospitalization in order to ensure that the rehabilitated person continues to be active. The patient should follow a properly designed home-maintenance program (physical, avocational, etc.) that incorporates proper body mechanics, relaxation, pacing, etc. These basic steps should become an integral part of the patient's daily routine, indefinitely, even if there is no pain.

Low Back Pain Management and the Role of Ergonomics   53

2. **Reengineering the work/home environment.** If the individual returns to the same poorly designed environment where, in many cases, he/she sustained the injury, there is a great possibility that reinjury may occur. Therefore, it becomes the task of the ergonomist to analyze and study the working or living environment (as well as the task) in order to ensure that the rehabilitated individual will be able to reengage in a productive lifestyle, while not being at risk of reinjury due to problems inherent in the environment.

METHODS OF ERGONOMIC INTERVENTIONS

At any of the three stages of the low back injury and its management process, ergonomics can intervene in the prevention and management of the problem through one or a combination of many strategies. Table 3.1 illustrates the elements of ergonomic interventions at the pre-injury, post-injury, and post-rehabilitation prevention stages. (It should be realized that these approaches are not stage-specific; that is, they may be applicable at any of the three stages of prevention). These intervention strategies can be grouped under at least six main areas. The principles and approaches to these intervention methods are described in Chapters 4–10.

1. Job analysis and design People, equipment, tasks, and job environments are studied and analyzed. Environments are engineered or reengineered to prevent accidents and control injury occurrence.

2. Postural and body mechanics interventions The results of job analysis are utilized to correct human work behaviors. Postural and body mechanics correction and practice are emphasized to ensure healthy alignment of the musculoskeletal system in order to reduce stresses while people are performing daily tasks.

3. Biomechanical approaches to stress reduction Biomechanical studies are used to augment the analysis of potential stresses on the human system (joints, muscles, ligaments) while it interacts with the external world.

4. Evaluation of human characteristics Human performance is evaluated through recognized methods of assessment of human abilities, in order to relate it to work ability or use it to aid clinical diagnosis and as a baseline for treatment efficacy.

5. Physical conditioning Active and passive forms of physical exercise and neuromuscular techniques—such as biofeedback, muscle reeducation, or functional electric stimulation (FES)—are designed and administered in order to allow individuals to achieve better control over body functions.

6. Work conditioning and work hardening Work capacities are increased and job simulation activities are used for vocational/avocational preparation in order to allow the individual to practice and refine work tasks under proper supervision. During this process, increasing people's awareness of their capabilities and limitations in reference to environmental demands becomes a primary interest in order to avoid reinjury.

4
Principles and Methods of Ergonomic Job Analysis and Workplace Design

The use of ergonomic knowledge in the analysis and design of jobs and tasks can have a significant impact on the reduction of work stresses and associated low back pain (LBP) problems. The objective of ergonomic job analysis (EJA) is to study the relationships among:

- job demands,
- environmental conditions, and
- human functional characteristics.

Job demands are obtained from a detailed analysis of the various tasks comprising the job, with the objective of matching task demands with human capacities required for successful job performance. The task demands are determined through direct observation and quantitative measurements of motion, time, forces, and sensory demands. To gain further information about task demands, interviews with the worker and the supervisor or employer are necessary.

The environmental setting and conditions in which the tasks are carried out are also assessed for their effect on task performance.

The human characteristics relevant to job performance are described in anatomical and physiological terms, as well as psychological aspects including aptitude, interest, temperament, and educational level. Collectively, they establish a human performance profile that determines functional capacities or abilities. The information obtained from the EJA is used to classify the job according to the demands of the work. The analysis is used to determine job duties a healthy person or an injured person can perform based on functional capacities (abilities) in relation to job demands. The analysis should take into consideration any environmental modification or other accommodations that the injured person may require to perform the job.

Systematic ways for implementation of EJA intervention programs are well documented and vary in complexity and generality (Abdel-Moty, Khalil, Diaz et al., 1991) (Abdel-Moty, Diaz et al., 1992). Job/task analysis and evaluation is a commonly employed technique in ergonomics. Job analysis can be done with the aid of motion and time studies; task analysis; and physiological and psychological tests employed by industrial engineers, psychologists, physiologists, and ergonomists. The analysis can be based on direct observation methods, work sampling analysis, computerized postural/motion analyses, electromyographic techniques, physiological measurements, psychophysical procedures for assessing perceived exertion, biomechanical analysis, cinematographic techniques, and force distribution measurements (Barnes, 1988; McCormick and Sanders, 1982; Chaffin and Andersson, 1984; Astrand, 1976; LeVeau, 1977; Grandjean, 1980, 1988). The level of the analysis varies from general to detailed descriptions of the individual's posture, body movements, and muscular exertion, as well as of the physical elements of the workplace. For patients with chronic LBP during rehabilitation, the following methods are suggested. The procedures described have been specifically developed in order to prepare the patient to reenter the competitive job market following rehabilitation.

METHODS OF ERGONOMIC JOB ANALYSIS

Ergonomic Job Analysis (evaluation and intervention methodologies) consists of four components.

1. Preliminary data collection
2. Initial evaluation
3. Intervention phase
4. Follow up evaluation

In the *Preliminary data collection* phase, and during the first week of patient's admission to treatment, an initial evaluation is performed in order to obtain both individual and job-related information. The components of this evaluation may include the following:

1. Basic biographic information and physical characteristics of the individual: age, weight, height, occupation, cause and course of injury, employment status, etc.

2. Qualitative description of the physical environment within which the job is performed. In this category the layout of the workplace and equipment parameters (locations, dimensions, priorities, frequency of use, etc.) are obtained through the patient's description and photographs of the work environment.

3. Patient's self-description of a *typical* work day. From this description, job tasks are identified, the average time required to perform each task is estimated, and the sequence of tasks performance is determined.

An *initial evaluation* can then be performed with the purpose of analyzing the patient's performance, especially muscular work. At this stage, the job (the physical environment as well as the task) is simulated and assessment is performed as follows:

1. Task/job simulation: The information gathered from the initial evaluation is used, in conjunction with the patient's input, to construct a workplace that closely simulates the actual workstation. It should be recognized that exact reproduction of the environment is impossible since there are many factors (heat, noise, fumes, etc.) that are difficult to emulate. As a matter of fact, an exact simulation of the workplace is not necessary. The goal here is to analyze patient's patterns of movement (body mechanics) within the environment.

2. Analysis of task performance: In order to evaluate the manner by which the patient performs job tasks, the patient performs tasks in the simulated environment that are similar to those encountered on the job. Emphasis should be on activities that are done repeatedly or for long periods of time. The goal is to identify the tasks that contribute more to stress production. For objective evaluation of performance, electrical activity of key muscles can be recorded (EMG). No feedback or suggestions for modifications or adjustments are to be given at this stage. The patient's self-report of discomfort/pain can be obtained at the beginning and end of this evaluation session.

3. Identification of the risk factors: While the simulated tasks are being performed, the evaluator should observe the patient's body mechanics and postural adjustment, identify critical motion patterns, and detect any mismatch between the patient's physical characteristics and the dimensions of the workplace. Also, levels of EMG activity are correlated with the different movements.

Following the identification of the risk factors, the *intervention phase* includes the following strategies:

1. Reengineering of the workplace: Sitting heights are adjusted based on anthropometric dimensions of the individual and work surface height; the layout of the workstation is modified so that all tools are within functional reach; additional equipment (for example, foot rest, keyboard holder, etc.) is recommended in order to compensate for major deficiencies. Expert system technology, such as Sitting Workplace Analysis and Design (SWAD), can be used to supplement the design and analysis process so that proper seating parameters are determined for the patient's anthropometric dimensions. The patient is then given detailed information about the rationale of the modifications made.

2. Postural adjustment: Provided that the physical match between the individual and the workplace is attained, the next step is to increase postural awareness. Principles of proper posture (Chapter 5) are implemented. It is important at this point to demonstrate to the patient, through EMG feedback, that these postural correction techniques do indeed reduce muscular tension and static stresses.

3. Body mechanics modification: Body movement at the workstation is corrected in order to minimize awkward patterns and reduce stresses resulting from activities such as twisting, over-reaching, and repetitive bending.

4. Learning and practicing: The patient is then given the opportunity to practice the new techniques and appreciate their efficacy in providing stress reduction. Simulations are repeated and body mechanics are refined. In large multidisciplincy rehabilitation facilities this type of activity is performed as a joint effort among several disciplines such as ergonomics, occupational therapy, vocational rehabilitation, and biofeedback. The patient reviews work activities, executes job tasks properly, receives suggestions for modifications or adjustments, and implements recommendations in the simulated environment. These activities assure the patient that he/she is capable of carrying them out when he/she returns to the actual work site.

A *follow-up evaluation* is then performed in order to determine, quantitatively, the changes in the outcome measures (EMG, self-report of pain, etc.) as a result of intervention. In a clinical setting this evaluation session may last 30 minutes.

ANALYSIS OF THE SITTING WORKPLACE

Every day people spend a great deal of their waking hours sitting on chairs and using office furniture that is poorly designed or improperly adjusted. A

Principles and Methods of Ergonomic Job Analysis and Workplace Design 59

poorly designed sitting environment can result in poor sitting habits, place undue stress on the musculoskeletal system and sensitive body tissues, be hazardous to health, and affect productivity. For those who already have pain, many studies have shown that there is a risk of increased back pain when they are required to sit for long periods of time. Mechanical stress on the lumbar spine was found to be 35% higher when sitting unsupported than when standing (Nachemson and Elfstrom, 1970). Several studies indicated increased risk of LBP for those who sit at work (Hult, 1954; Kroemer and Robinette, 1969; Magora, 1972; Andersson et al., 1984). These stresses are basically static in nature and usually are manifested as neck and shoulder pain, headaches, upper and lower back discomfort, muscle fatigue, and leg pain and numbness. In order to minimize these stresses, experts have defined two basic goals.

1. Proper healthy alignment of the musculoskeletal system while sitting
2. Proper design and adjustment of the workplace (tools and tasks)

There is a large number of human and environmental variables that are encountered when seated workplaces are designed (Fig. 4.1). The multitude of these variables has led to the establishment of guidelines for proper design of the seated workplace. These guidelines are well established in ergonomic technical literature. With the advent of ergonomics, chairs are becoming precision sitting machines that are functionally correct and scientifically accurate for the specifics of the job. For individuals with pain, an adjustable

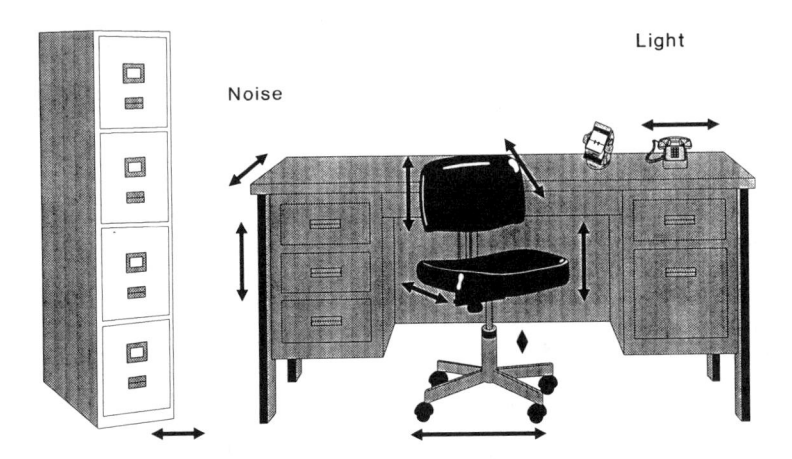

FIGURE 4.1. The seated workplace has many design and environmental parameters that have to be considered when fitting people to the task. Adjustability permits matching the work environment to the characteristics of the workplace user.

TABLE 4.1 Guidelines for the Design of Seated Workplaces

General
- Work tools should be accessible and kept within the functional reach of the operator.
- Stresses can develop if the head is too far forward or backward during desk activities. Excessive bending, twisting, and reaching are related to the onset of pain and discomfort.
- Different types of work require different work surface heights for comfort and optimal performance. Light detailed work, such as writing, requires a work surface close to the elbow height of the seated person, provided there is enough clearance under the work surface for the knees and legs.
- Reach requirements of the task sometimes cause nonneutral postures. Severe deviation from neutral postures occur when work tools are placed outside comfortable reaches.

Chair
Seat and Backrest
- The back and seat supports should be contoured to the body to provide maximum support without interfering with circulation in the muscles.
- The chair should be upholstered with slightly porous, rough-textured material to dissipate heat, facilitate circulation, reduce static pressure, and support the body.
- Adjustment for tilting the seat and backrest is important to allow for better support.
- Adjustment of the seat and the backrest should be independent. The angle between the seat and backrest should be more than 90° (ANSI, 1988). Torso-to-thigh angle less than 90° leads to great spinal stress and may lead to fatigue and discomfort (Grandjean, 1988). As this angle is increased work tasks and tools should be readjusted accordingly to avoid incorrect posture.

Backrest
- If it is possible to provide a high backrest for office work, it would be preferable since most people often wish to lean back (Grandjean, 1988). A high backrest supports the trunk more than a small backrest.
- The backrest should be angled about 10–15° from vertical. Back angle helps minimize stress on spinal structures and maintain the spine/leg relationship. The height of the backrest should provide adequate cervical and head support. The backrest should be concave to the front at its top to support the head.
- Short backrests should support the lumbar region of the spine and should not interfere with free arm movement if used as a secretarial chair.

Seat
- The seat height should be easily adjustable to allow the feet to rest on the floor or on a footrest while maintaining correct work surface height, knee angle, and support for the lower leg. If the seat is too high, legs will dangle, increasing pressure on the underside of the thigh and encouraging sliding. This will not allow the individual to use upper back support. If the seat is too low, elbows will be raised, increasing static tension in cervical musculature.
- Adjustable seat depth is desirable to allow correct thigh support and proper knee clearance and avoid pressure on the back side of the lower leg (calf area).
- The front edge of the chair should not exert pressure on the thighs or calves and impair circulation.
- Chair height and inadequate support under the feet can result in stresses due to cutting off circulation at the thighs and to the individual's inability to use the backrest while sitting.
- Seat width should allow the seated person to move about and assume various postures.

Principles and Methods of Ergonomic Job Analysis and Workplace Design 61

TABLE 4.1 *(Continued)*

Arm Rest
- The weight of the arms is supported, in part, by the musculature of the neck and upper back. Prolonged sitting or standing to perform simple tasks while the elbows are unsupported imposes continuous static stresses on the cervical muscles causing muscle fatigue and pain. Therefore, it is desirable to provide adjustable arm support while not interfering with the individual's performance at the workstation and without interfering with musculoskeletal functions.

Others
- Depending on task demands and floor surface condition, casters are desirable and can give greater freedom of movement. They ease ingress/egress movement with the workstation (ANSI, 1988).
- Five-spur pedestal are preferred for stability, balance, safety, and ease of movement.
- Provide swivel chairs to avoid excessive torsional moments in seated workplaces.
- Chairs that provide half-sitting–half-kneeling posture are no better than conventional chairs and could be worse than a well-designed office seat (Drury and Francher, 1985; Grandjean, 1988).

chair should allow adequate, natural, comfortable, and flexible support and stability for body segments (elbows, lumbar region, upper back, legs, and the head), as well as distribution of body weight and freedom of movement. A *good* chair can add as much as 40 productive minutes to the working day of each individual (Tichauer, 1979). Well designed chairs are a prerequisite to the safety and health of seated workers, including those with preexisting injury. A well-designed chair will favorably affect posture, circulation, the amount of effort required to maintain posture, and the amount of strain on the spine (Andersson et al., 1986).

The guidelines for the design of workplaces for seated operators are summarized in Table 4.1 and are illustrated in Figures 4.2 through 4.6.

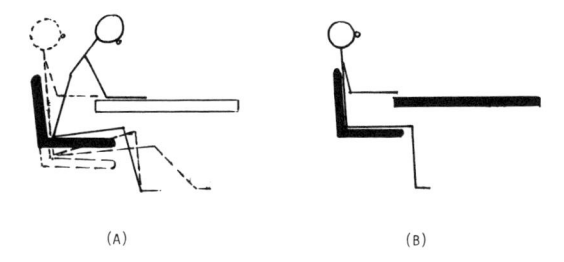

FIGURE 4.2. (A) A tall person given a low desk forces bending over the work; thus creating stress at the neck and back. An attempt to lower the chair will create stresses at the shoulders and discomfort for the legs. (B) Ideal match where the work surface is approximately at elbow level.

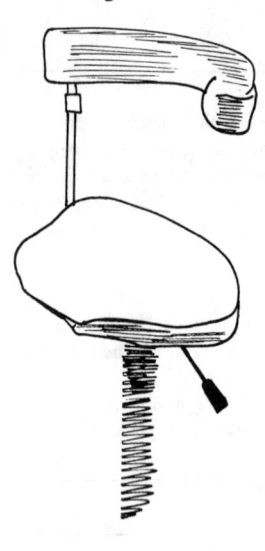

FIGURE 4.3. A chair with frontal support is useful for tasks requiring forward hand and trunk activities such as that of a dental assistant (Khalil, 1974).

WORKING WITH VISUAL DISPLAY TERMINALS

Visual display terminals (VDTs) are becoming a dominant piece of office equipment, secondary only to the telephone. The wide use of VDTs and personal computers in office automation has created situations in which the operator's eyes are oftentimes *glued* to the VDT screen. Computer operators are sometimes required to sit for long periods of time in order to perform tasks such as data entry, data retrieval, programming, and word processing.

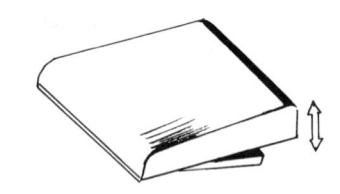

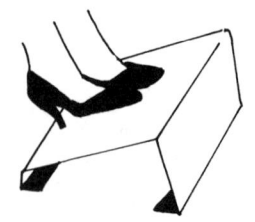

FIGURE 4.4. Many types of footrests are available; some of which are adjustable. These devices are useful in ameliorating differences beween inidiviual anthropometric dimensions and existing workplace furniture in order to achieve an ergonomically correct and healthy posture.

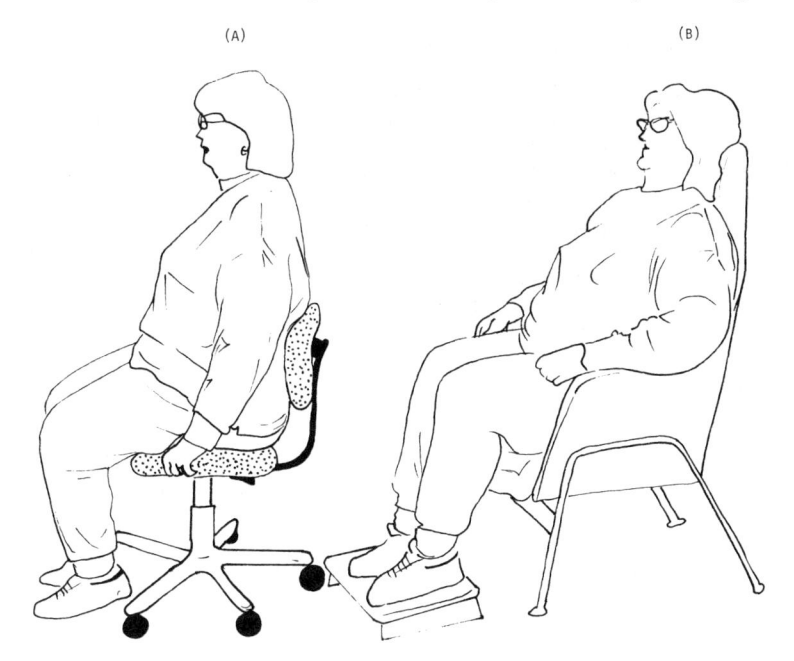

Principles and Methods of Ergonomic Job Analysis and Workplace Design   63

FIGURE 4.5.   A well-designed chair for office work (A) is not suitable for relaxed sitting of this individual. A traditional chair and an adjusted environment provide better support and comfort (B).

With a VDT screen, the eyes remain in a rather narrow range with respect to the screen. It is always desirable that the operator be able to scan—mainly within the range of vision and with minimum head and neck movement—the screen, the keyboard, and the source document. This depends upon three interrelated factors: 1) viewing distance, 2) viewing angle, and 3) *visual-ability* of the operator. Considerations and guidelines in designing VDT workplaces are summarized in Table 4.2 and Figures 4.7 and 4.8.

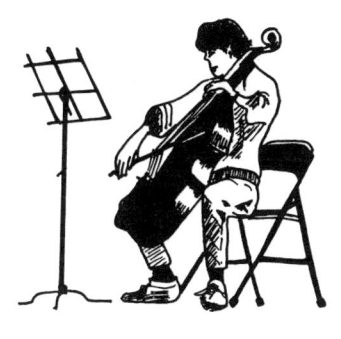

FIGURE 4.6.   An example of a task and a chair that are incompatible. The person does not make use of the backrest and seat edge cuts circulation of the thigh muscles.

TABLE 4.2 Considerations in VDT Workplaces

- Proper viewing distance and angle are a function of the visual attributes of the operator. Use of visual correction, such as regular (or bifocal) eyeglasses or contact lens, has to be recognized in the design and adjustment procedure.
- VDT screen should be within 5–10° below and horizontal. This angle can be maintained for long periods of time with minimum discomfort. Deviation from this angle will result in rapid muscle fatigue and potential neck and shoulder discomfort.
- Entire primary viewing area (top of screen to keyboard to source material) should be less than 60° below the horizontal plane passing through the eyes (ANSI, 1988).
- Relative placement of the source documents, the keyboard, and a reflection-free screen should provide better eye-hand coordination and less strain on the neck and shoulders.
- The keyboard should fall directly below the hands with the elbow at 90°. An independent adjustable support surface for the keyboard is preferred. If the keyboard support is not adjustable, chair height should be adjusted so as not to violate elbow height requirement (elbow angle should be about 90°).
- In situations where the job requires a combination of keypunching, answering the telephone, and/or writing, the placement of the different work elements and possible use of a telephone headset becomes critical.
- Resting the palms and forearms gently is recommended for long-term keyboard use, in order to support the weight of the upper extremity and allow shoulders and neck muscles to relax during work. The chair's armrest could be useful. Shoulder, elbow, and wrist joints should be maintained in a rather neutral position.
- Having a stand for reference material is essential to reduce neckache. By positioning the document holder at screen level, one-third of the movement is eliminated. This way the user can easily avoid unnecessary eye, neck, and head movement. The position of the document holder should be alternated from one side to the other in order to avoid localization of stress.
- The workstation desktop should have two levels: one for the monitor and another for the keyboard. The levels should be independently adjustable to suit the user's comfort. The range of adjustment should be based on anthropometric data and on the relative height of the seat and the keyboard. In a VDT workstation, the essential element in determining the height of the work surface is the keyboard height.
- The parameters of the chair's seat and backrest should be considered in order to provide back stability and relaxation of the back muscles, to prevent static pressure on sensitive body tissue. Chair dimensions must be personalized and reevaluated for each individual on the basis of certain aspects of function and surface anatomy (Tichauer, 1979). The backrest should provide comfortable support. High back support is restful for the neck and trunk muscles, at least during rest periods. It is always desirable to minimize static pressure by eliminating pressure points that can impede blood circulation, allowing more even distribution of body weight on the seat.
- The angle between the upper arm and forearm should not exceed 135°, otherwise muscular effort to support the arm will increase and may result in fatigue and discomfort (ANSI, 1988).

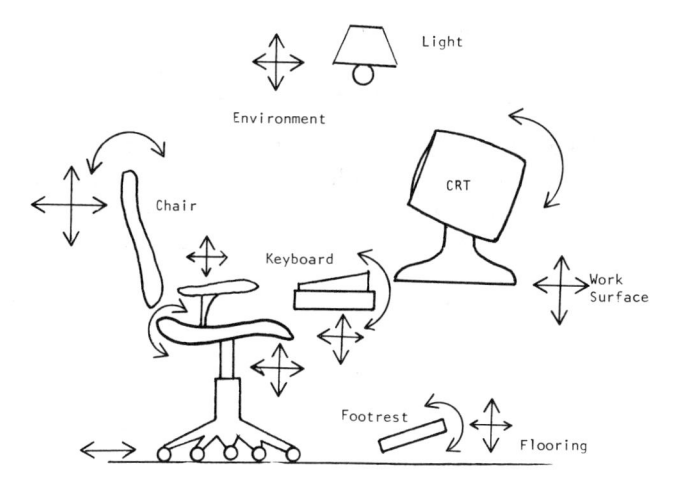

FIGURE 4.7. Adjustability permits a better match between an individual's anthropometric dimensions and his/her workplace.

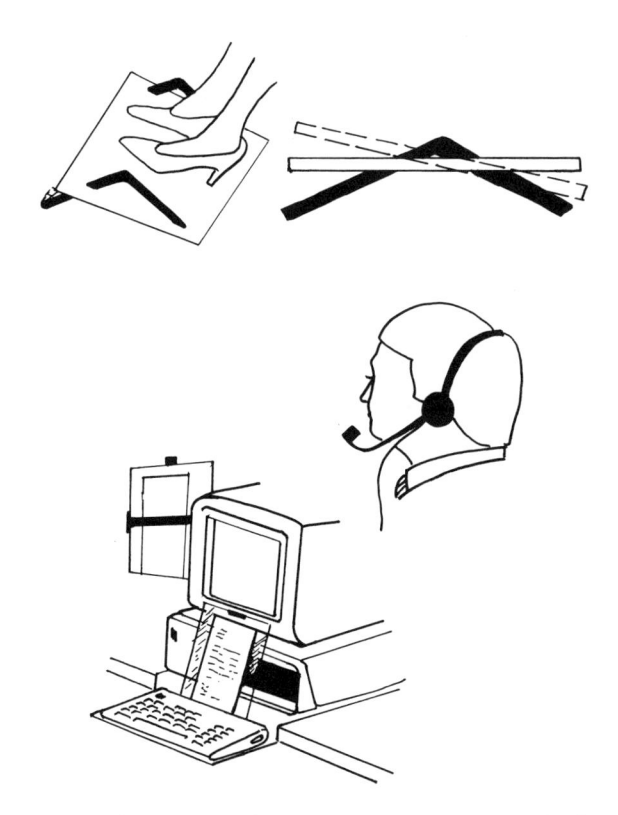

FIGURE 4.8. Examples of ergonomically inspired designs that help alleviate musculoskeletal stresses.

COMPUTER-AIDED WORKPLACE DESIGN

In order to facilitate the implementation of ergonomic principles and guidelines in workplace design, computer-aided design (expert system technology) can be used. An *expert system* is a form of artificial intelligence where an intelligent software uses knowledge and inference procedures to solve problems that require human expertise.

Computer-aided design represents a new direction in the implementation of ergonomic knowledge through the use of microcomputer and expert system technology. With computer-aided design and expert systems, workplaces are designed and/or analyzed and proper seating devices are determined for the individual who is using the workplace in a very simple, yet professional, manner. Expert systems make ergonomic guidelines for the design of sitting workplaces available to the consumer and interested groups.

Sitting workplace analysis and design (SWAD) is an example of such expert system technology applied to ergonomics and workplace design (Abdel-Moty and Khalil, 1986a, 1986b, 1987a, 1987b, 1988b, 1988c, 1989).

TABLE 4.3 SWAD Output when Designing a *New* VDT Sitting Workplace*

Parameter	Dimension
Chair	
Back support	
Vertical length	28.8
Horizontal width	11.7
Angle of inclination	−10°
Seat	
Height (top to floor)	17.4
Breadth (side to side)	17.9
Depth (front to rear)	17.0
Elbow rest height of chair (seat to top)	9.0
Work Surface	
Height (top to floor)	26.6
Minimum restrained reach (normal area)	7.9
Maximum reach (maximum area)	18.1
VDT	
Mid-VDT height	15° below 42.8
(depending on the distance from table edge)	
Keyboard base height (to floor)	25.1
Knee clearance height	2.0
Footrest height	3.0

*Examples of individualized workplace dimensions obtained from the Expert System "SWAD." These dimensions are slightly adjusted in the workplace to meet practical environmental considerations and constraints.

Principles and Methods of Ergonomic Job Analysis and Workplace Design 67

The computer algorithm combines inputted static and functional anthropometric data of the individual with ergonomic principles and guidelines to produce an optimal sitting workplace. The SWAD model is a comprehensive, practical, interactive, easy-to-use expert system. It is designed to facilitate the design and analysis of sitting workplaces. The usefulness of this microcomputer-based model was examined through actual applications. Through SWAD's menu, the user can

- design a new sitting workplace, or
- study and analyze an existing one.

If the user's aim is to design a new sitting workplace, the system collects descriptions of the different work tools that will possibly be used in the new environment. If the user requires an analysis of an existing facility, the system inquires about dimensions, parameters, and features of the existing workplace. SWAD then simulates the workplace through computer graphics. The second step is to review the information provided by the user in order to analyze the current workplace or to design a new one. The major function in this step is to identify the tasks performed by the seated worker and to model or remodel the layout of the work area to reduce stress on the human body. Knowledge about the existing work environment, which is supplied by the user, is checked against the rules. SWAD then provides the user with physical stress analysis and potential stress points due to the existing workplace. Samples of SWAD's screens are presented in Tables 4.4 and 4.5 as well as in Figures 4.9 through 4.13.

TABLE 4.4 SWAD in the Analysis of an Existing Workplace (actual dimensions) and Recommendations for its Modification (optimal dimensions)*

Parameter	Actual Dimension	Optimal Dimension
Chair		
Backrest length	20.0	25.0
Backrest width	21.0	>8.6
Seat height	18.5	18.5
Seat depth	18.5	15.5
Seat breadth	21.0	20.0
Desk		
Height	30.0	28.5
Width	66.0	>43.5
Depth	30.0	>21.7
Knee clearance	6.0	2.5
Footrest height	0.0	3.0

*All dimensions are in inches.

TABLE 4.5   Important General Ergonomic Considerations in the Design of Workplaces

- It takes little effort to make a workstation comfortable and less stressful.
- Design for safety.
- Design to accommodate population percentiles. Do not design for an average person.
- Consider the population from which the measurements were taken and for which the design is to be made.
- For space requirements, accommodate the large person.
- For reaches, accommodate the small person.
- Provide adequate space for movement.
- Consider the limits of muscular force and strength.
- Educate and train workers.
- Design flexible workstations that can adapt and change according to the postures and habits of different people.
- Individualize the selection of appropriate seating to meet the dimensions of the individual and the demands of the task.
- Design tools to facilitate task performance.
- Lay out work areas within normal easy access reaches (horizontal as well as vertical).
- Have a special place to do each job so that equipment and supplies are always ready for immediate use.
- Locate control switches within easy reach.
- Tools should be positioned properly. All work tools should be placed within easy reach of the individual and stored in a convenient location.
- Design workplaces at which tasks can be conducted either sitting or standing.
- Select work surface and chair heights appropriate for the individual and the task.
- Take note of visual attributes of the individual.
- Raise the work surface for fine or precise work and lower it for heavy work.
- Provide good light (intensity, quality, brightness, contrast), good ventilation, and control other environmental conditions.
- Load stress (several tasks to perform) and speed stress (high work pace) are undesirable, particularly when combined with environmental stresses.

```
          Input/Output Menu

    1. Enter Biographic Data and
       Anthropometric Dimensions.
    2. Enter Job Description.
    3. Analyze/Design a Regular S.W.P.
    4. Analyze/Design a VDT S.W.P.
    5. Reset Parameters and
       Return to Main Menu.

       Enter Your Choice: ■
```

FIGURE 4.9.   Computer printout of SWAD's input/output screen.

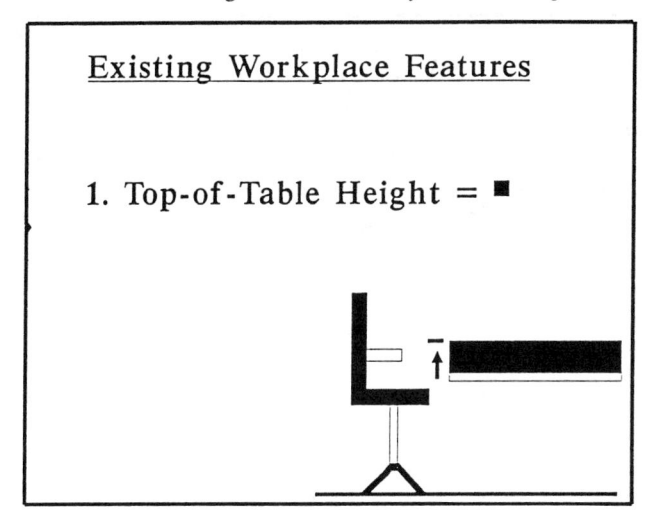

Principles and Methods of Ergonomic Job Analysis and Workplace Design   69

FIGURE 4.10. In the analysis of an existing facility, SWAD requests the parameters of the current workplace: as in this example, the height of the table top.

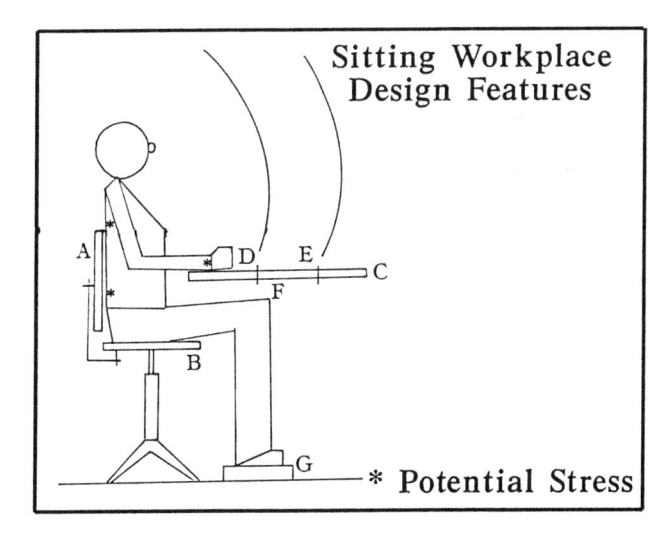

FIGURE 4.11. A sample printout of SWAD's output screen showing a regular sitting workplace. An * indicates that the current workplace parameters are likely to place stress at that body part.

70   Ergonomics in Back Pain

Recommended Workplace Layout

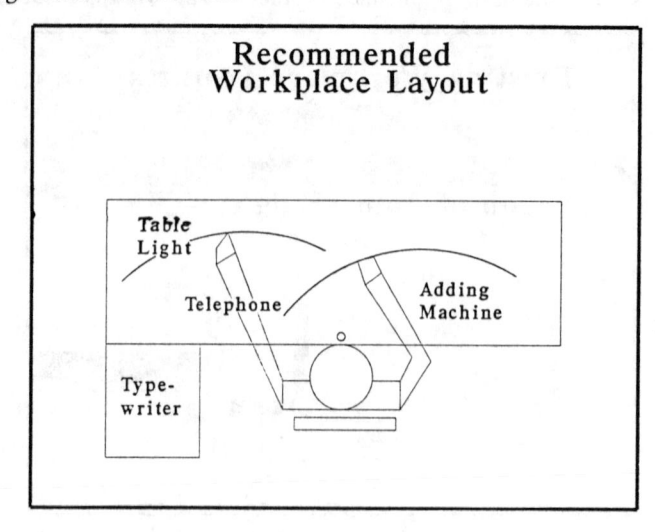

Table Light
Telephone
Adding Machine
Typewriter

FIGURE 4.12.   A sample printout of SWAD output of a recommended layout.

WORKPLACE DIMENSIONS

NOTE: All dimensions are in inches.
   Use figure to identify parameters A, B, C, etc.

Chair parameters:
  A. Back support parameters:
    Vertical length   18.6
    Horizontal width   15.1
    Angle of inclination $-10\frac{1}{2}$ from the vertical
  B. Seat height (top of seat to floor)   15.7
    Seat breadth (side-to-side)   17.9
    Seat depth (front-to-back)   17
    Elbow rest (seat-to-floor)   9
  C. Work surface height (top-to-floor)   26.6
  D. Minimum restrained reach (normal area)   7.9
  E. Maximum reach (maximum area)   18.1
    Mid VDT screen height   15 degrees below 40.6
    (depending on distance from edge of the table)
    Keyboard base height (to floor)   23.9
  F. Knee clearance   2.0
  G. Foot rest vertical height   0

Prepared by:

Date:

FIGURE 4.13.   A sample printout of SWAD output of the suggested quantitative parameters describing the work environment.

GENERAL GUIDELINES FOR WORKPLACE DESIGN

In the design of general workplaces, be it in industry or at home, ergonomic guidelines should be considered together with basic principles of engineering design. Table 4.5 provides important applicable guidelines. Figures 4.14 through 4.16 illustrate the use of anthropometric dimensions in designing optimal workspaces to minimize stress. Complete discussion of all the information and guidelines for the design of systems, facilities, equipment, and products for human use are beyond the scope of this book and can be found in Woodsen (1981.)

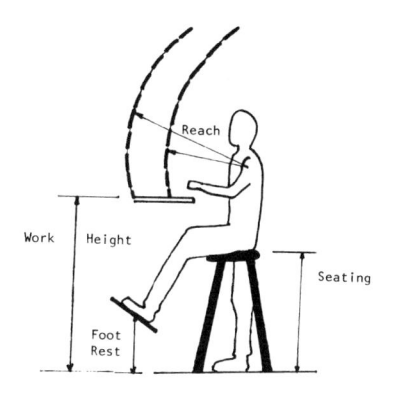

FIGURE 4.14. Ergonomics offer many guidelines and design principles for the sit/stand workplace. These can be found in the technical literature (e.g. Woodson, 1981). Workplaces allowing alternating sitting and standing are very common in industry and the set of recommendations for such environment is far more complex than for seated workplaces.

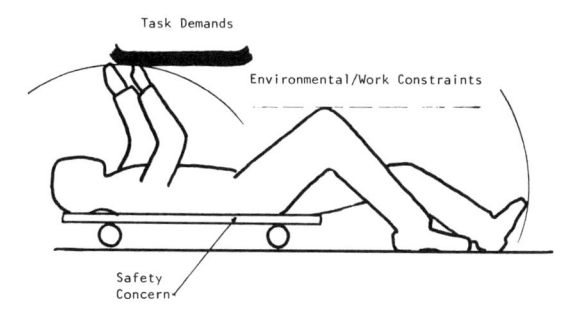

FIGURE 4.15. There are several design and safety guidelines to deal with working in confined spaces. In such instances, use of body mechanics and postural principles should be carefully examined for the individual situation. The technical ergonomic literature should be consulted for design and safety guidelines.

72   Ergonomics in Back Pain

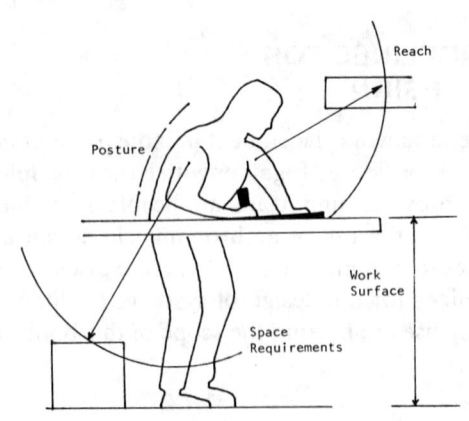

FIGURE 4.16. Ergonomic guidelines for the design of standing workplaces are numerous. These take into account individual, task, and environmental differences. While many of the guidelines for seated workplace may still apply, standing workplaces require special considerations (Woodson, 1981).

5
Principles and Methods of Interventions Through Postural Correction

There is a definite relationship between good posture and good health. Good posture is achieved through alignment of the musculoskeletal system and all its joints in its neutral, balanced position. The neutral position is that position where the least amount of stress and/or energy expenditure is needed to maintain the position. It is the position from which movements can be made with good facility. In standing posture in the anatomical position, the head and spine are balanced in relation to the line of gravity (Fig. 5.1).

ANATOMICAL PLANES OF REFERENCE

As shown in Figure 5.1, the anatomical position is defined when the body is in a static standing erect position with the upper limbs extending at the sides and the hands in position of supination (palms out). In describing posture in space, the body can be divided into segments by means of imaginary planes cutting through it (Fig. 5.2). The coronal or frontal plane is a vertical plane passing through the body from side to side, dividing it into ventral and dorsal segments or front and back segments. The saggital plane is a vertical plane passing through the body in an anterior-posterior direction. It divides the body into symmetrical right and left halves. The transverse plane is a plane that divides the body into upper and lower segments. Starting from the

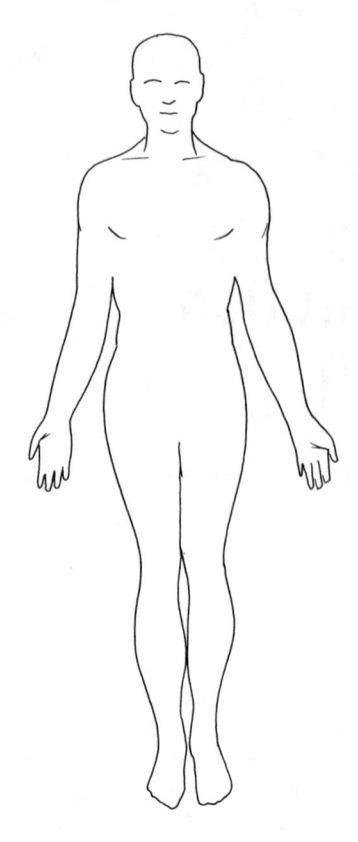

FIGURE 5.1. The anatomical posture.

anatomical position, movements (extension, flexion, abduction, adduction, and rotation) can be defined and described in reference to one or more of these planes. The anatomical positions permit most joints to start movement from natural neutral positions.

POSTURE AND HEALTH

The keys to good posture are proper body mechanics, exercise, self-awareness, and proper design of tools and equipment. Poor, awkward postures cause fatigue, strain, and eventually pain, and should be corrected. Deviation from neutral positions usually result in poor posture. Poor posture may result in structural deformation of the body, muscular contractures, pain in the back and legs, decreased lung capacity, poor circulation, intravascular pressure, kinks in the bowel, and many irregularities in the

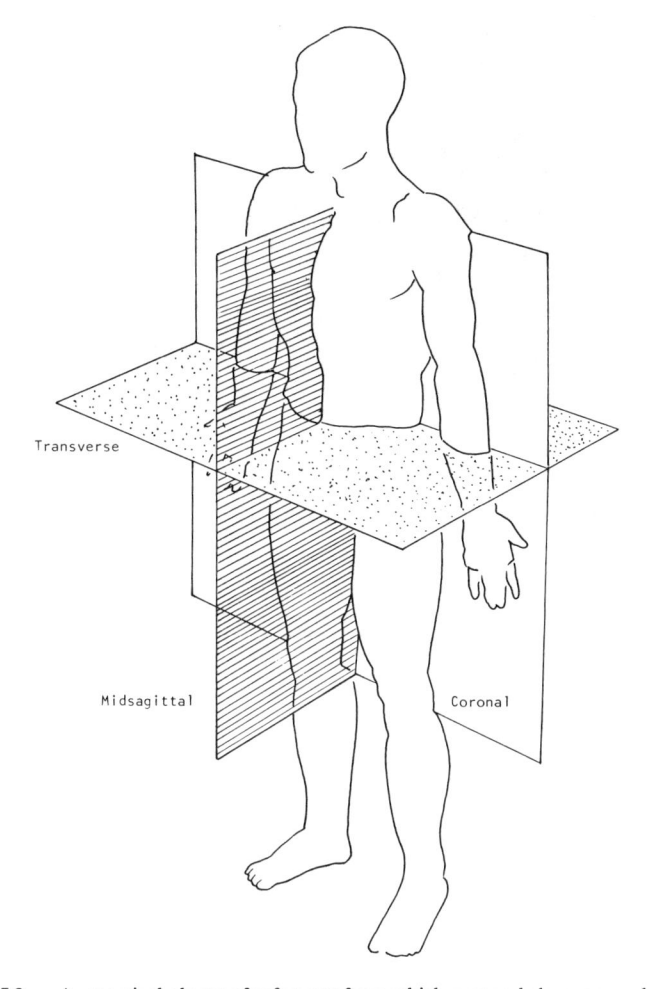

FIGURE 5.2. Anatomical planes of reference from which postural changes can be defined.

functions of the body. Poor posture can also cause loss of stability, falls, slips, and other related accidents. Faulty posture and poor alignment of the musculoskeletal system develop slowly and may not be observed by the individual. Poor posture can develop due to obesity, weakened muscles, emotional tension, and poor postural habits.

Figures 5.3 through 5.7 illustrate examples of postures that are considered biomechanically poor for various reasons. These range from poor postural habits to poor design of the workplace.

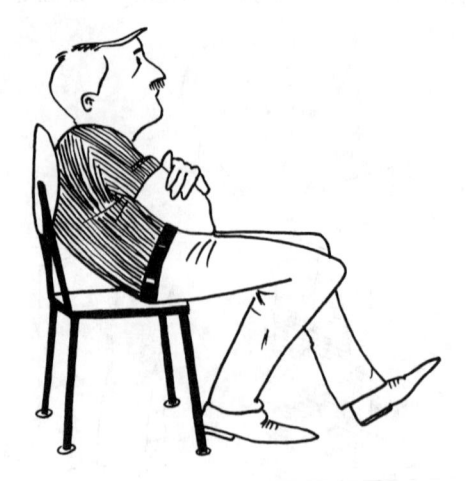

FIGURE 5.3. Poor posture: slouching in a chair creates biomechanical imbalance in the musculoskeletal system and may lead to low back pain.

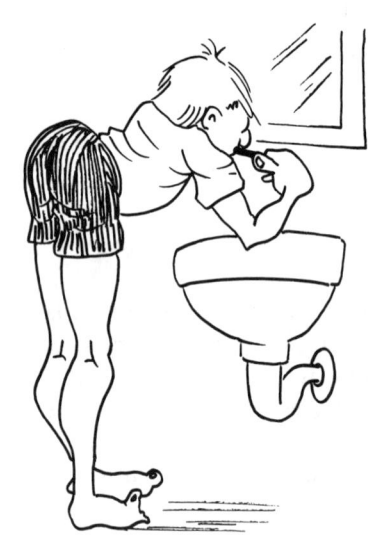

FIGURE 5.4. Maintaining good posture should be practiced in all daily activities in order to avoid cumulative stresses.

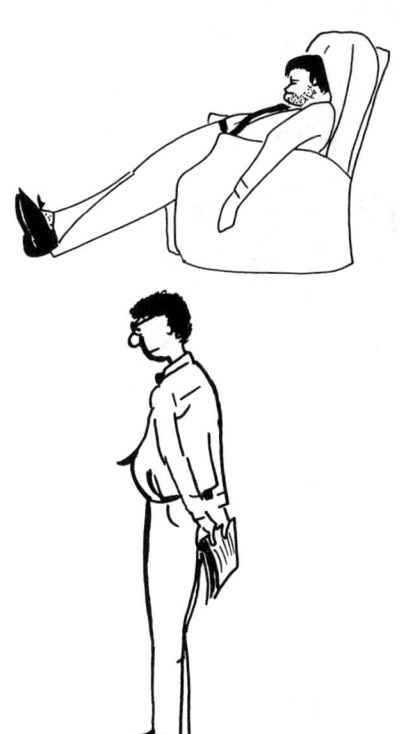

FIGURE 5.5. Faulty postures may feel comfortable because they relax the muscles. However, they can be very stressful if maintained for long periods and should be corrected.

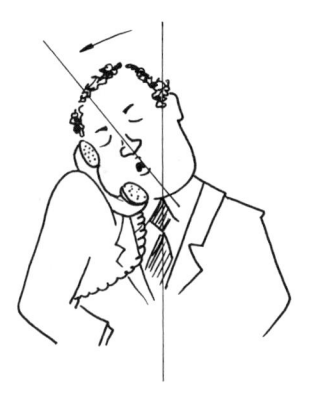

FIGURE 5.6. An example of a simple task that is commonly performed improperly. Such posture should be avoided. In addition to stressing the neck and shoulders, extreme deviation of the head from the neutral position creates unequal mechanical loading on the spine.

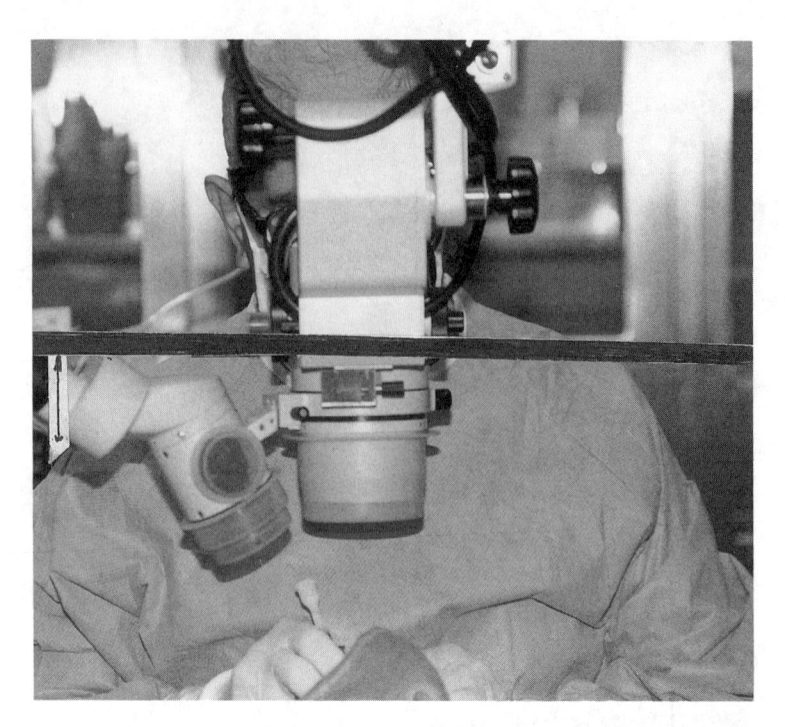

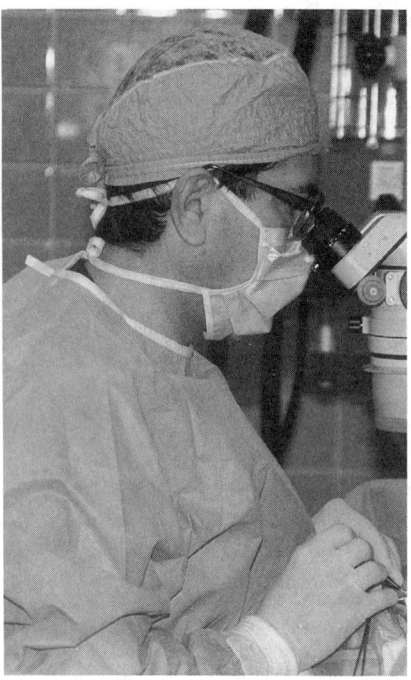

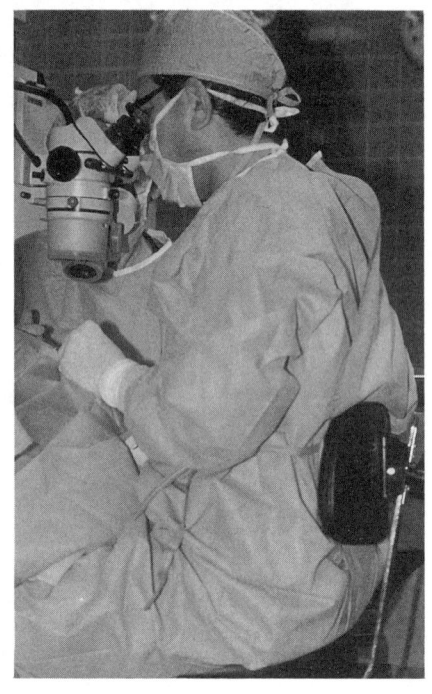

FIGURE 5.7. Uneven shoulders, forward flexion, and poor neck postures are commonly seen in the operating room. An eye surgeon performs in this static, stressful posture. Adjustment of the chair and equipment is important to relieve the stress.

PRINCIPLES RELATED TO POSTURE

The center of gravity is the imaginary point representing the weight center of an object. In the human body, each component (bones, muscles, etc.) has a center of gravity; each segment (arms, forearms, hands) has an aggregate center of gravity; and the whole body has a combined center of gravity (CG), where the entire weight of the body is concentrated and all parts exactly balance (Fig. 5.8 and 5.9). For the purpose of stability the line of gravity (the vertical line passing through the CG) should fall inside the base of support (example: the feet). The lower the position of the CG, the more stable the body is. In the anatomical position, each segment of the body is balanced vertically on the segment beneath it and the line of gravity passes between the feet (in the middle of the base of support). If the distribution of body weight is uneven, or if a load is carried, the line of gravity will shift position, putting more demand on the muscles (Fig. 5.10). The body will compensate for the load by bending to the opposite side of the load to bring the line of gravity again inside the base of support.

Human posture is maintained by muscles. Muscles that maintain the general upright posture, such as the muscles of the back (trapezius and latissimus dorsi) are strong. It is believed that normal posture is maintained through reflex behavior. A good posture requires normal muscular tone. If smaller, nonpostural muscles are used to maintain posture or balance of the body, increased stress and fatigue will result.

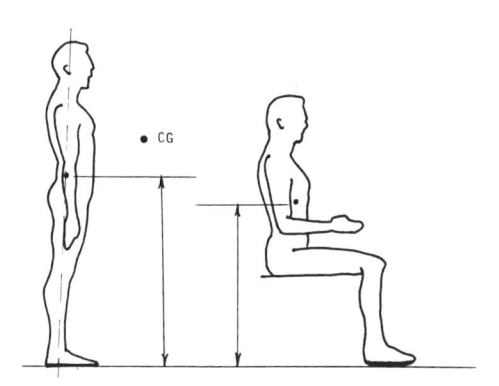

FIGURE 5.8. The anatomical posture: The body is well balanced; the line of gravity falls within the base of support. The position of the center of gravity of neutral standing and a sitting posture are shown.

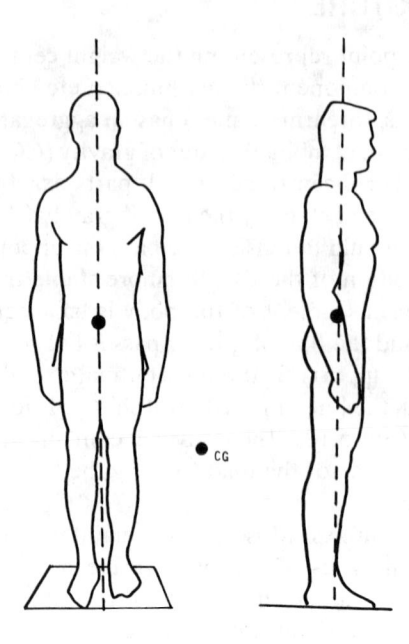

FIGURE 5.9. Center of gravity in relation to the line of gravity in the standing posture.

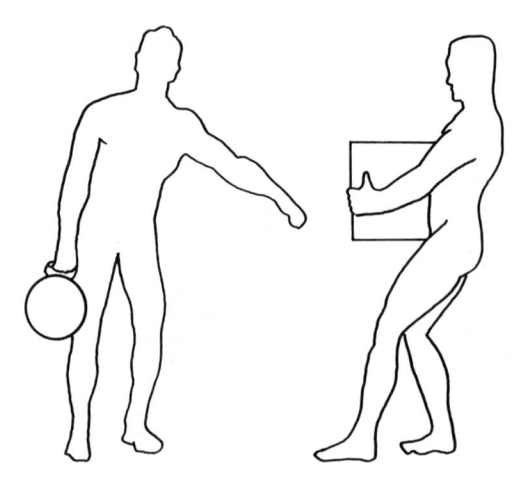

FIGURE 5.10. Postural adjustment automatically centers the total mass of the body and the object over the base of support in order to maintain body balance.

POSTURE AND ENERGY DEMAND

Good posture is less energy demanding. However, a posture requiring a minimum of energy expenditure does not necessarily fulfill the requirement of good posture. The energy cost of a task depends on the amount of muscular activity involved in the task. More effort is used in sitting than in lying; more effort is used in standing than in sitting; and more effort is used to support an awkward posture than a neutral one. Since the energy cost of standing is more than in sitting, and both of them are more than in lying, sitting has always been preferred by ergonomists over standing. This is predicated on the following facts:

TABLE 5.1 Guidelines for Good Posture

- Maintain head, neck, and back as close to the same coronal plane as possible.
- Keep joints in their neutral position. Frequent use of extreme joint position is fatiguing.
- Use equipment and tools that enforce proper posture.
- Provide a wide and balanced base of support at the feet while standing.
- Avoid prolonged periods of static posture. Static posture causes problems in muscles, joints, and blood circulation. Prolonged periods of static posture reduce body efficiency.
- Use postures giving best mechanical advantage for the muscles used.
- Stand straight without slumping.
- Alternate sides of the body to prevent localization and concentration of stress on one side and to prevent fatigue.
- Sitting is better than standing. However, a workplace permitting both sitting and standing is preferred. Whether sitting or standing, provide enough space to allow freedom of movement and change in posture.
- Support the arms and the back while sitting.
- Don't hunch trunk over your desk.
- Don't slouch when reading in a chair.
- When on the telephone, use headset or support elbow on desk top to keep neck aligned. Switch sides periodically.
- Analyze posture to pinpoint what is causing pain and discomfort.
- Practice perfect posture while standing, sitting, or moving.
- Reclined postures are acceptable, if the chair provides adequate support of the head and if the task is readjusted within the viewing area.
- People who wear bifocals, trifocals, or "half-eyes" have reduced effective range of viewing and should avoid awkward positioning of the head.
- Don't promote only one posture since this can lead to static muscle loading and fatigue. Allow for movement.
- Maintain the knees at a level equal to or slightly higher than that of the hips, which enables you to use the backrest, allows alignment of spinal structures while sitting, and prevents impeding circulation to the thighs from seat edges.
- Weight should be distributed uniformly under the thighs while sitting, and under the feet while standing, to ensure proper balanced support of the spine, head, and shoulders.

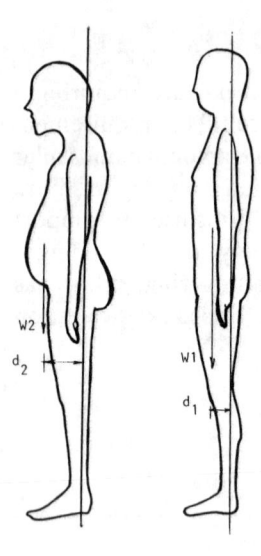

FIGURE 5.11. Good posture and physical fitness help reduce static loading on the lower back [(W1*d1) is less than (W2*d2), where "W" is body weight and "d" is the distance to L5/S1].

1. Less energy is consumed in a seated posture, thus delaying or avoiding fatigue.

2. Sitting frees the legs for other operations (for example, foot controls).

3. Biomechanical stresses on the lower extremity are reduced.

4. Blood circulation is easier, provided that no circulation restriction is imposed by equipment used.

5. Better body balance is maintained.

6. There is less chance of assuming a wrong posture.

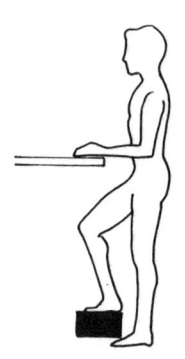

FIGURE 5.12. Standing for long periods of time creates stress on the back muscles, causing back pain. One way to relieve stress is to alternate putting one foot on a short stool.

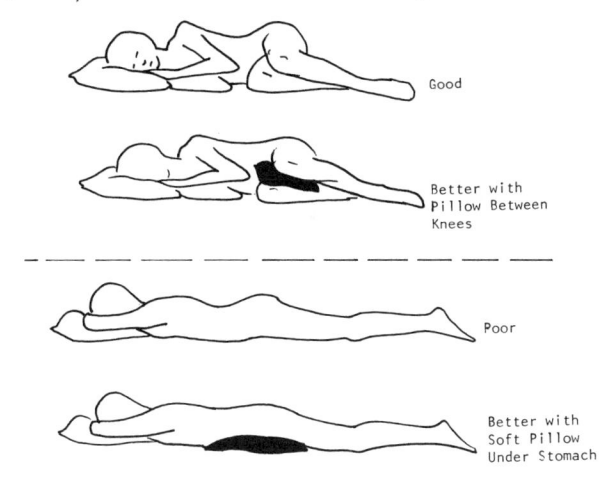

Principles and Methods of Interventions Through Postural Correction 83

FIGURE 5.13. Examples of poor and good sleeping postures.

Assuming proper posture in the seated position is extremely important. Although relaxed posture requires less energy consumption, it might cause undesirable pressure on the inner organs. Proper sitting posture can be achieved through the use of well-designed seats and backrests. On the other hand, long periods of sitting are considered undesirable because

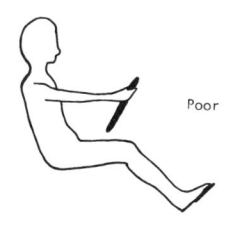

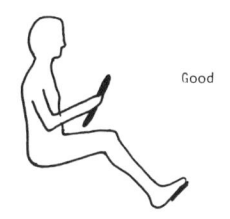

FIGURE 5.14. Poor and good driving postures.

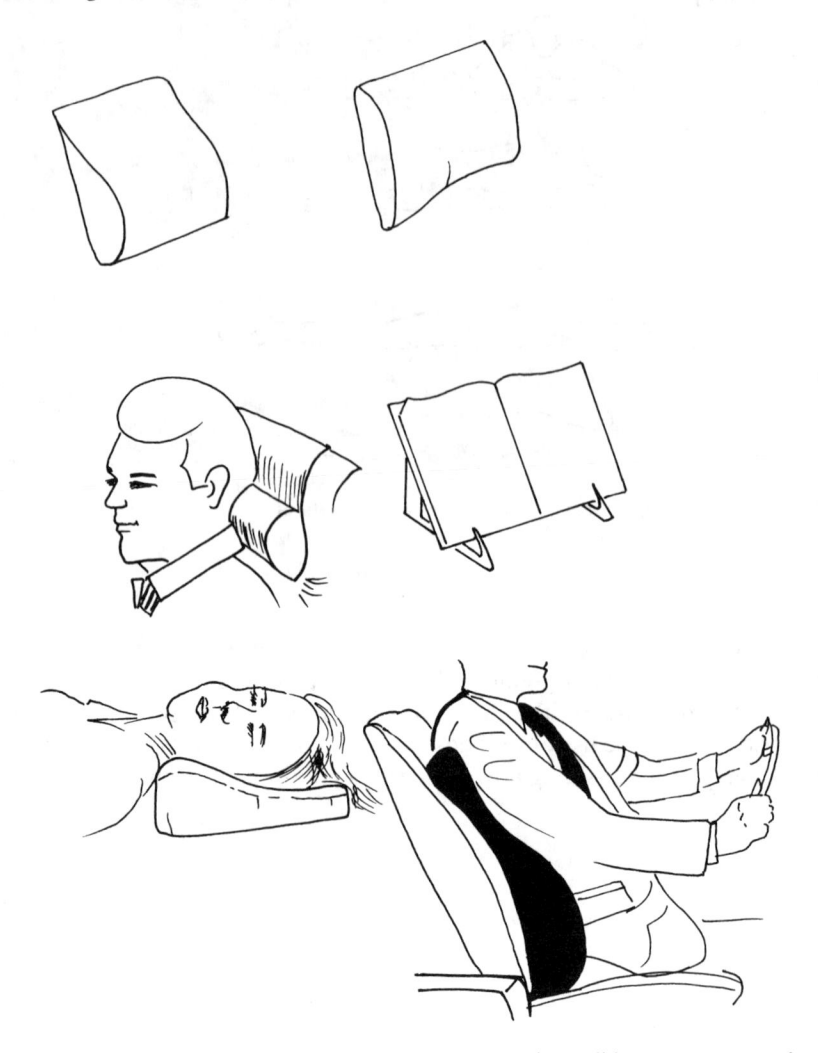

FIGURE 5.15. Posture control aids may be useful in certain conditions to correct poorly designed or improperly adjusted equipment and furniture.

- they may lead to slackening of muscles;
- low energy consumption and lack of exercise accompany long periods of sitting, which may interfere with blood circulation or cause muscular atrophy;
- round back may develop;
- if seats and backrests are not well designed, they may cause cramping, static stress, and cutting off of circulation.

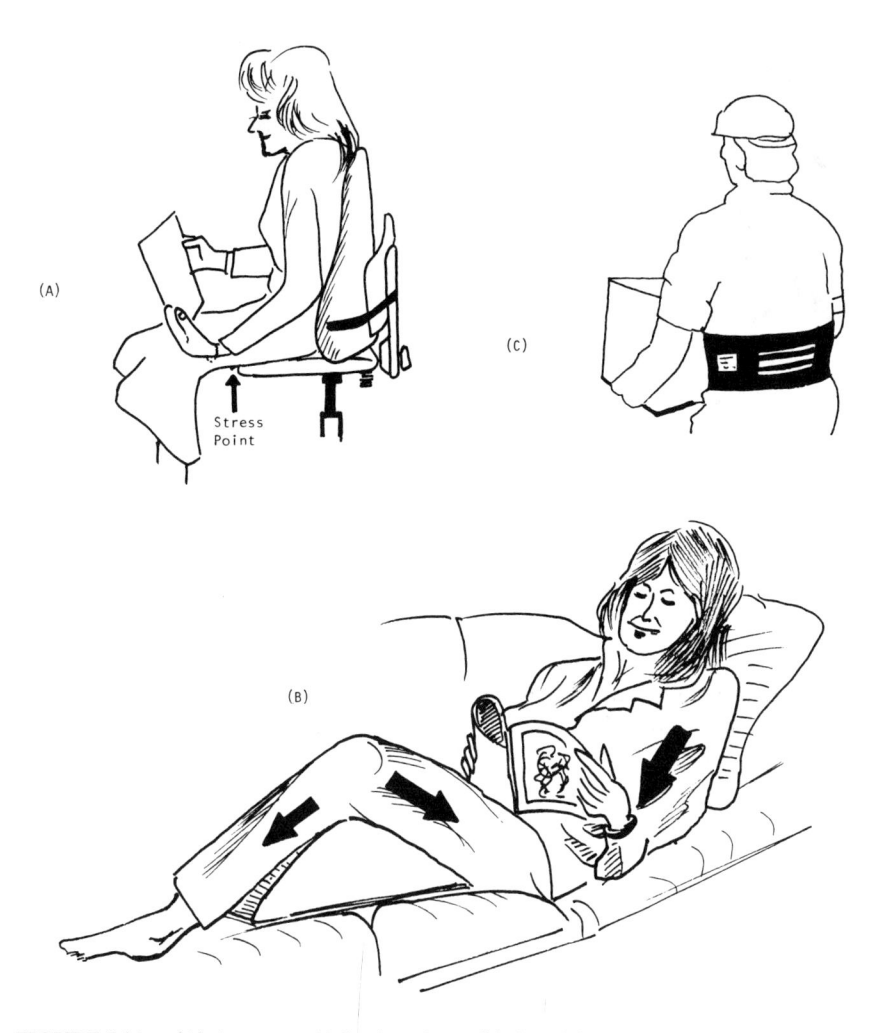

FIGURE 5.16. (A) A posture aid that interferes with the original design of the chair may relieve stress on the back but may create stress underneath the legs. (B) Proper use of pillows can help achieve a biomechanically comfortable and relaxing posture. (C) The use of back belts has become popular. No research universally supports the use of belts to prevent back injury. Some evidence even suggests that, while belts can serve as a reminder, they may weaken muscles and cause deconditioning. Belts do not substitute ergonomic comprehensive solutions to workplace stresses.

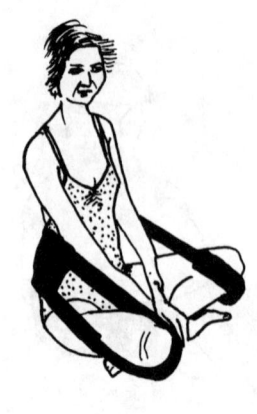

FIGURE 5.17. Nada chair™—a product used to support the back while seated in the posture shown. Such aid is useful for short duration. Long-time use may irritate the knees and hips.

Some operations require standing because

- better access to the work area is provided;
- greater force capacity is available; and
- walking is easier from standing.

In general, alternating between sitting and standing is better than sitting all the time. Table 5.1 provides general ergonomic guidelines for good posture. Figures 5.11 through 5.17 illustrate some of these principles.

6
Principles and Methods of Interventions Through Biomechanical Approaches to Stress Reduction

Biomechanics is an interdisciplinary field of study that integrates knowledge from the biological sciences and engineering mechanics. Formally it has been defined by the American National Standards Institute (ANSI, 1988) as "The study of the human body as a system operating under two sets of laws: the laws of Newtonian mechanics and the biological laws of life." Occupational biomechanics as a subset of the general field of biomechanics provides greater emphasis on the working environment. This includes the design of tools, equipment, and work spaces to reduce mechanical stresses on the body for optimum use and comfort. Occupational biomechanics provides the biomechanical basis for ergonomics and concentrates more on the effects of stress, motion forces, and responses to these. Its applications span a wide range of human activities including rehabilitation, engineering design, sports, industrial operations, and activities around the home.

In discussing biomechanical intervention, one might be able to appreciate the value and rationale of the methodologies by understanding the basic biomechanical principles of the human system.

THE LEVER SYSTEM ACTION

In order to accomplish movement of the body, the muscles use the skeletal system bones as lever arms and the joints as fulcrums. The lever action

88   Ergonomics in Back Pain

provides several mechanical advantages suited to body functions. There are three classes of levers.

First-Class Lever

The first-class lever occurs when the fulcrum falls between the resistance and the effort. An example of this in the body is that of a raised head (Fig. 6.1). The front of the head is the resistance, the occipital-atlanto joint is the fulcrum, and the muscles of the back of the head provide the effort. This type of lever is well suited for balancing.

Second-Class Lever

The second-class lever occurs when the resistance falls between the fulcrum and the effort. The closest situation to this type is standing on one's toes (Fig. 6.2). There are very few examples of second-class levers in the musculoskeletal system—although the body uses this type of lever in the form of tools, such as the wheelbarrow.

FIGURE 6.1.   First-class lever.

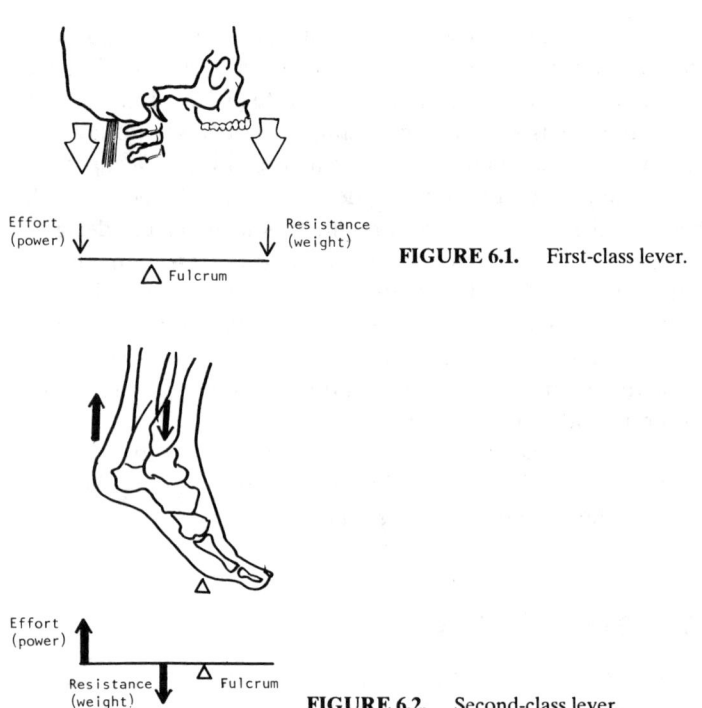

FIGURE 6.2.   Second-class lever.

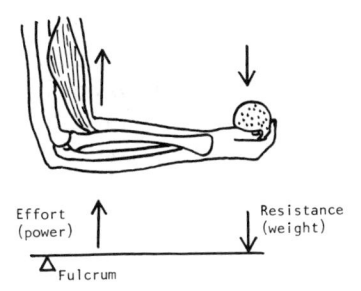

FIGURE 6.3. Third-class lever.

Third-Class Lever

In the third-class lever the effort falls between the fulcrum and the resistance. This type of lever is well suited for rapid, delicate movements. It requires that effort be greater than resistance. An example of this is flexing the forearm. Most of the levers in the musculoskeletal system are of this class. An example of this class of levers is given in Figure 6.3.

MECHANICAL ADVANTAGES OF LEVERS

The advantage of levers is derived from the relation:

Effort (power) × Effort Arm = Resistance (weight) × Resistance Arm

In first-class levers a small force can be made to overcome a larger counterforce. In third-class levers, distance moved by the point where the weight is applied is more than the distance moved by the point where power is applied, and a larger effort is needed to move a resistance. However, this sacrifice enhances mobility and reaches.

BIOMECHANICAL MODELS

Biomechanical models are used to predict the severity of the stresses associated with specific tasks. Biomechanical models use information concerning body segment parameters (weight, length, mass, center of gravity), body posture parameters (angles between links), and the external load demand to determine the stress forces on body components. These models consider the body as being made up of rigid links joined at articulations and moved by musculature. Tasks are analyzed biomechanically through determination of forces, angles, velocities, and acceleration at each joint. Estimates of inertial forces and reactive moments can also be calculated. This approach assists in predicting the body's response to the task being performed by identifying the stresses imposed on the musculoskeletal system. Biomechanical models are appropriate for nonfatigue states of performance. When fatigue becomes a factor, biomechanical models need to be combined with electromyographic techniques and measurements of other physiological responses (for example, heart rate).

Static and dynamic biomechanical models have been developed (Ayoub and El-Bassoussi, 1978; Morris et al., 1961; Nachemson and Elfstrom, 1970; Armstrong, 1965; Chaffin, 1969b; Schultz et al., 1982; Anderson et al., 1985; Garg and Chaffin, 1975; Khalil and Ramadan, 1987). An example of a simplified static biomechanical model is given here for illustration (Fig. 6.4A). The model is constructed to calculate the amount of stress placed on the lower back when a person is lifting an object. Many back injury problems occur at the lumbo-sacral region of the spine, which is considered the weakest link in the back. In order to calculate the amount of stress placed on the musculoskeletal system or on specific components of the system, such as the fifth lumbar–first sacral (L5/S1) disk space, a three-link model can be used (Fig. 6.4B). This model has the advantage of being simple and quick in providing a rough

(A) Simple Lifting Task

(B) 3-Link Biomechanical Model

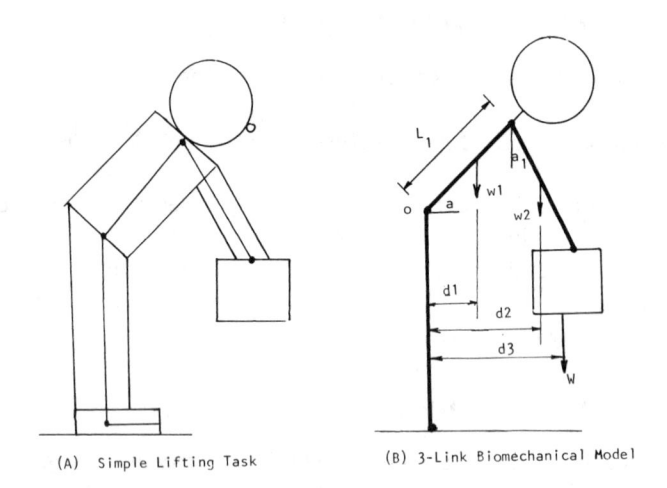

FIGURE 6.4. (A) One type of biomechanical modeling approaches in which the body was defined in terms of three links, each describing a part of the body while permorming a static lifting task (B) Torque around point "o" can be calculated as:

$T_o = (W1 \times d1) + (W2 \times d2) + (W \times d3)$

if: $L_1 = 36"$, arm length = 20", angle a = a1 = 45°, w = 10 lb, w2 = 3 lb, w1 = 100 lb, d1 = 5", d2 = 10", and d3 = 20"; then it can be shown that T_o will be 1682 lb. in.

approximation of the amount of stress placed on the back. However, it lacks the anatomical accuracy and faithful representation of the real system.

One can also resort to a more complex five-link model (Fig. 6.5). This model is usually computerized to facilitate calculations while changing the posture parameters. The simplicity or complexity of a model is determined by the objectives of the model, the effects desired, and the costs available to develop such a model. To calculate the magnitude of forces on various body joints, Khalil and Ramadan (1987) model the human body as a two-dimensional, eight-link system representing movement around seven joints: ankle, knee, hip, L5/S1, shoulder, elbow, and wrist (Fig. 6.6). Considering the trunk

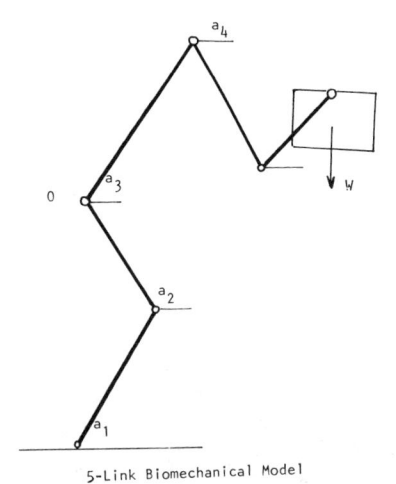

FIGURE 6.5. A more complex biomechanical model in which the body was defined in terms of five links and six joints. (Khalil and Ramadan, 1987).

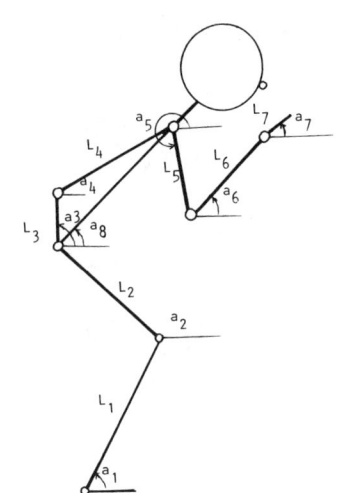

FIGURE 6.6. A multilink computerized biomechanical model of an individual performing a simulated lifting task.

as two links allows for the calculation of stresses at the back muscles and the L5/S1 junction. The posture is defined by angles between body links and the horizontal. When the posture changes (which implies changing joint angles) the magnitude of stresses also changes (Fig. 6.7). Values obtained for force can be compared to strength limits of the disk, vertebrae, ligaments, and muscles (NIOSH, 1981; Chaffin, 1969b).

It should be recognized that most back injuries occur during dynamic tasks (tasks involving movement). Dynamic biomechanical models are needed to evaluate stress in such cases. A dynamic task would produce added stresses that, in combination with the load carried and the posture assumed, could expose an individual to a high risk factor. A comparison between the biomechanical stresses generated in static and dynamic tasks for the same load is shown in Figure 6.8 (Khalil and Ramadan, 1987). The most stressful posture occurs quite early after the lifting action has started. Maximum compressive forces generated from the dynamic model are higher than those obtained from the static model, except at the beginning, middle, and end of the lifting action. This equality is because the acceleration is zero at these points. As the velocity of the body increases so do the stresses generated on the back.

Biomechanical models can also be used for the analysis of job tasks (Khalil, Asfour, Marchette, Omachonu, 1987). In rehabilitation, biomechanical models can be used for:

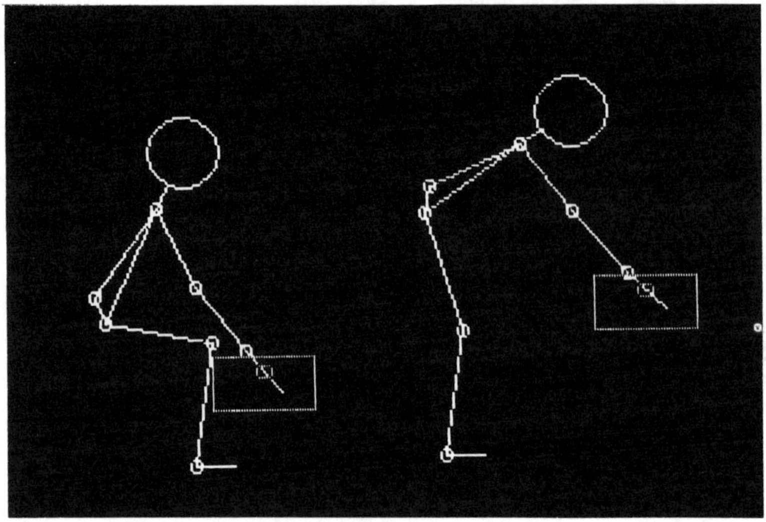

FIGURE 6.7. Using biomechanical models, stresses on the back and joints can be calculated for the different postures assumed by a person, taking into consideration the weight and configuration of the load handled.

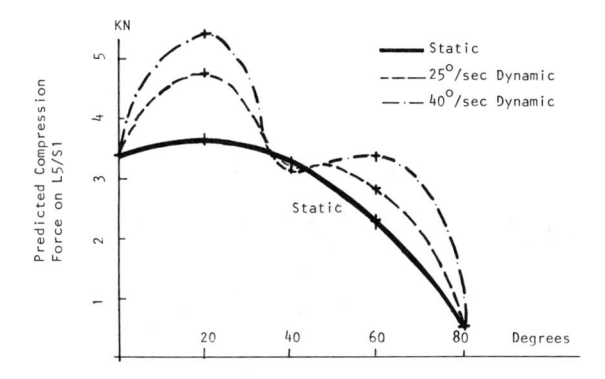

FIGURE 6.8. Trunk angle (from horizontal) versus predicted L5/S1 force for various modes of activity: static and dynamic and two speeds. The calculated compression force decreases as the angle of forward flexion of the trunk increases. Forces due to the dynamic task at 40°/sec induced higher compressive force. All force approached same value at 40° of flexion (Khalil and Ramadan, 1987).

- determination of the forces acting on the body in various postures;
- recommendations on engineering and task designs in order to reduce stresses when performing a task;
- education of patients in the use of proper body mechanics;
- analysis of sports and other activities.

7
Principles and Methods of Interventions Through Knowledge and Awareness of Body Mechanics

Intervention through body mechanics (also known as posture in motion) implies the use of the optimum ways to sit, stand, lift, carry, squat, climb stairs, and perform other activities of daily living. There are numerous advantages of using proper body mechanics in activities of daily living. Improper use of body mechanics taxes the body's soft and hard tissue and leads to poor alignment, faulty posture, fatigue, and pain.

COMPATIBLE AND NONCOMPATIBLE MOVEMENTS

The structure and function of the skeletal, muscular, and nervous systems determine the compatibility of movements. For example, forearm flexion and supination are compatible because both movements use the bicep muscle, which is capable of performing both actions with ease. However, hand pronation and flexion performed simultaneously represent noncompatible movements. To work against the natural capabilities of the muscle is stressing. If a series of noncompatible movements are necessary, then the action is fatiguing, painful if continued, inaccurate, and weak. It is imperative that comfortable ranges and nonstressing compatible movements be understood so they can be applied at the practical performance level. Other examples of noncompatible movements include wrist deviation and holding or hand pronation and pulling.

Principles and Methods of Interventions   95

BODY MECHANICS IN LIFTING

The number of injuries due to lifting and manual handling of heavy weights is alarming. Guidelines to limit the amount of weight lifted have been recommended. Even though there is no guarantee that the use of such

TABLE 7.1   The GOLDEN RULES in Handling Objects

1. Think...
   - What is to be lifted?
   - Is it ready to be moved?
   - Where does it go?
   - Is the pathway clear of hazards?
   - Is the destination ready to take the load?
2. Examine...
   - Check for sharp corners.
   - Check for any nails, loose handles, splinters, or burrs.
   - Use gloves or splash aprons if needed.
   - Use foot protection and safety glasses if required.
   - Do you need help?
3. Get Set...
   - Set the feet firmly.
   - Place one foot alongside or as close as possible to load.
   - Place other foot slightly behind the load.
4. Get a Grip...
   - Grasp object by handles or in a firm grip with *both* hands.
5. Get Ready...
   - Choose the technique that feels the most comfortable.
   - Try to keep the object balanced between both hands.
   - Set muscles of legs, torso, shoulders, and arms to lift.
   - LIFT...
   - Keep load close to the body.
6. Go...Smoothly...
   - Lift gradually.
   - Avoid jerky motions.
7. Follow Your Feet...
   - Move with your legs not with the body.
   - Watch your footing.
8. Use Your Head...
   - Put the load down in the reverse order of lifting.
   - Avoid overreaching while unloading.
   - Avoid unbalancing the load.
   - Get help or mechanical aid.
   - Do not overestimate your power.
   - If load slips from your grasp GET CLEAR. Don't catch it.
   - Don't lift over critical equipment.

TABLE 7.2 General Guidelines for Body Mechanics

- Work within viewing area.
- Bring objects close to your focus without crouching.
- Stimulate blood flow and reduce stress by moving and shifting weight. Don't sit in one spot.
- Rest elbows at a level so that the telephone receiver is at ear level.
- Don't hold the telephone between the head and the shoulder.
- Don't carry too much in one hand. Redistribute the load or use a backpack.
- When pulling, switch hands to avoid straining muscles.
- Free hands for taking notes or dialing the telephone by using speaker phone, using a headset, or installing a padded shoulder rest.
- Avoid prolonged hyperextension and hyperflexion when showering, shaving, etc.
- Use both hands to work symmetrically and in smooth path of motions.
- When carrying or lifting, keep load as close to the body as possible.
- Slide—don't lift or carry.
- Avoid holding against gravity.
- Get as close to the work area as possible, while maintaining proper posture and freedom of movement.
- Avoid twisting and sudden turning. Turn the whole body as a unit. Point both feet in the direction of movement.
- Avoid abrupt reflex movement.
- Avoid repetitive movements.
- Avoid working over your head level for extended periods of time.
- Minimize overreaching, as well as reaching behind the head. Keep forward reach short.
- Use ballistic movements at the joints.
- Motions of the trunk that are performed often should be kept well within the trunk ranges of motion.
- Make use of stronger muscles to perform the same task.
- Modify sleeping habits or reevaluate bed and pillows.
- Exercise for stretching and strengthening.
- Driving requires less effort when you are in the proper position. Sit with the shoulders level with the steering wheel. Adjust side and rearview mirrors so that you don't have to turn your head to use them.
- When lifting, place feet far enough apart for stability.
- Test (size) the weight before handling it. If heavy don't hesitate to ask for help. Use mechanical help (trolley) whenever possible.

guidelines will completely prevent or reduce incidence of low back injury, these guidelines are looked on favorably. The National Institute of Occupational Safety and Health (NIOSH, 1981, Chaffin and Andersson, 1984) presented these guidelines in its effort to reduce stresses and thus control injuries to the musculoskeletal system due to lifting. NIOSH's guide considers a lifting task as "…. the act of manually grasping and raising an object of definable size without mechanical aid. The duration of such an act is normally less than two seconds, and thus little sustained exertion is required." The

Principles and Methods of Interventions 97

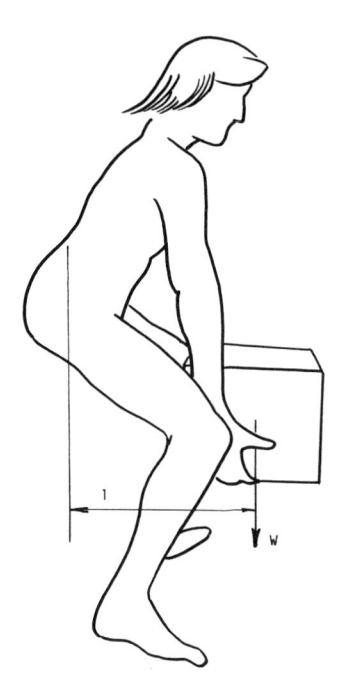

FIGURE 7.1. Important parameters in lifting include body posture, object size and weight (w) and distance of weight away from body (l).

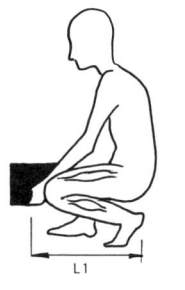

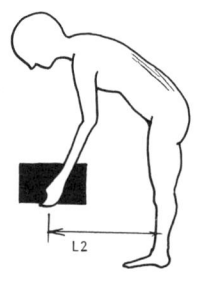

FIGURE 7.2. Proper body mechanics calls for avoiding lifting objects away from the body by bringing the object as close as possible to the body (L1 < L2). Whenever possible, guidelines recommend the use of the strong leg muscles to perform the lifting instead of the weaker back muscle.

98   Ergonomics in Back Pain

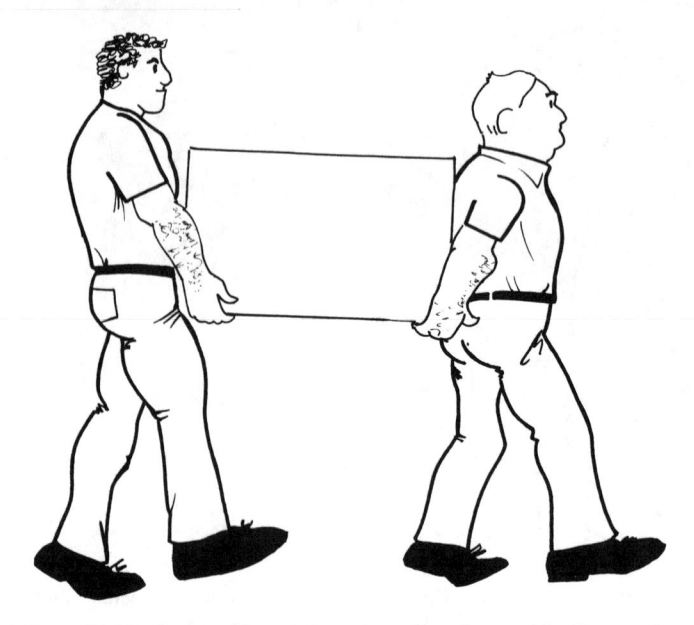

FIGURE 7.3.   Seeking help to lift an awkward or a large/heavy object is a good practice. Coordinating the lifting and carrying functions with the partners is another safe practice.

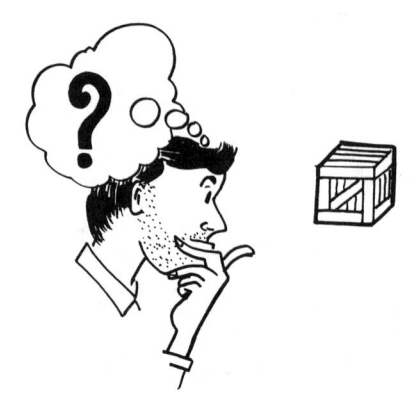

FIGURE 7.4.   Think before attempting to lift, and concentrate on the task while performing it.

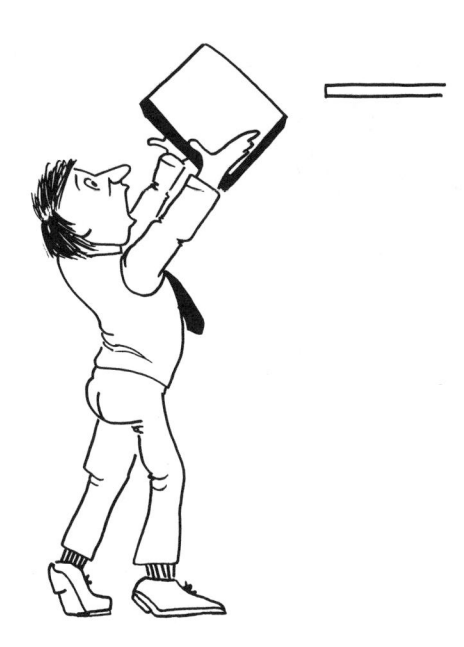

FIGURE 7.5. Avoid overhead lifting to extreme heights.

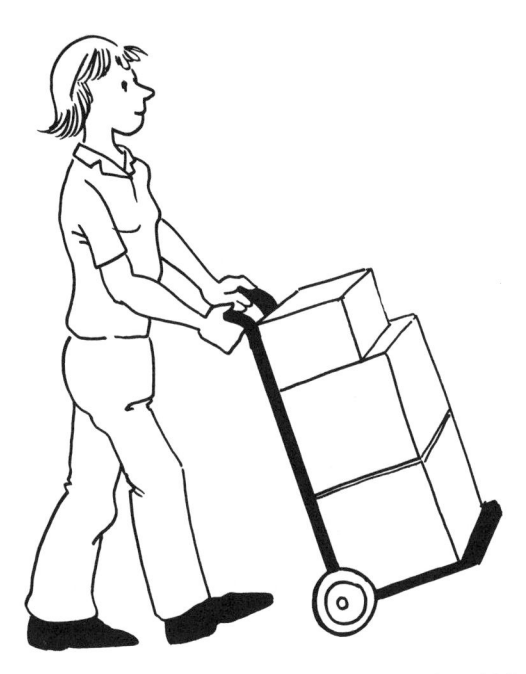

FIGURE 7.6. Mechanical aids are recommended whenever possible. Maintain good upright posture during pushing and pulling activities.

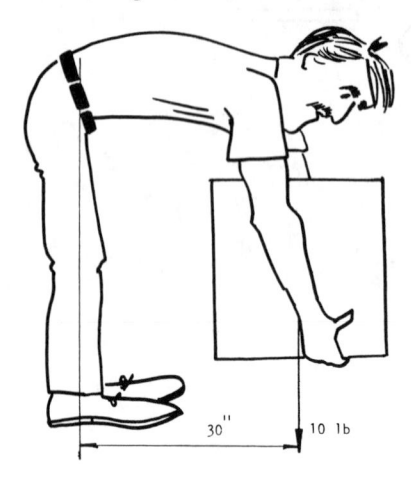

FIGURE 7.7. A box weighing 10 pounds produces about 300 inch-pound of torque on the low back structure if handled as shown. Added to this are the stresses imposed by the body's own weight in that posture. These stresses are significantly less when proper body mechanics are employed.

determination of lifting limits in the guide was based on the following set of assumptions and variables:

1. Lifting is done smoothly.
2. Lifting is two handed and symmetric.
3. The object lifted is of moderate width.
4. Lifting technique is unrestricted.
5. There are good handles, shoes, floors, etc.
6. Favorable environmental conditions exist.
7. There is no fatigue factor.
8. The individual is physically fit.

These assumptions limit the applicability of the recommended limits, since most lifting tasks in industry or in regular daily tasks are performed under different sets of conditions. It should be indicated that the values recommended by NIOSH fall mostly below what workers are required to do on the actual job and in many work situations. These values do not take into account the large variations in strength and lifting capabilities among individuals, males and females, people of various age groups, etc. However, these guidelines are the most commonly recognized recommendations for designing and evaluating lifting tasks in industry. NIOSH has been revising the 1981 guide, but the revised edition has not been officially released as of the time of preparation of this manuscript. Readers are advised to contact NIOSH directly for a copy of the new guide.

Tables 7.1 and 7.2 summarize the rules and guidelines of proper body mechanics for lifting and various activities of daily living. Figures 7.1 through 7.7 illustrate some of these principles.

8
Principles and Methods of Interventions Through the Evaluation of Human Characteristics

Recognition of human characteristics is essential for establishing capacities, capabilities, and limitations of individuals. These are the prerequisites of determining human performance profiles; for designing tasks, equipment, and environments; for determining disability; and for evaluating the efficacy of treatment or rehabilitation. In the area of objective evaluation of human performance, physical, physiological, functional, and activity-related responses can be measured. Collectively, these measurements can establish a quantitative profile of performance abilities of individuals. The evaluation of human performance is the scientific assessment of human characteristics at a certain point in time (time of evaluation). The main objectives of human performance assessment are:

- to provide an accurate description of the individual's characteristics;
- to translate findings of physical, physiological, behavioral, and functional abilities into performance potential for daily tasks, including work;
- to suggest or eliminate occupational assignments for individuals if the physical abilities and the demands of the task do not match.

Human characteristics can be expressed in terms of human capacities or human abilities. *Human capacities*, which may also be referred to as tolerance levels, represent the limits of the anatomical, physiological, and psychological systems of the individual. These capacities are dependent on hereditary factors, gender, age, physique, and other individual variables. *Human abilities* are human capacities modified by individual behavioral attitudes as well as by external factors, including injuries, pain, and environmental or social stressors (Fig. 8.1). Theoretically, for a healthy motivated individual, capacities and abilities should be equal under the same environmental conditions.

The concepts of human performance analysis are a cornerstone of the science of ergonomics. When these concepts were introduced in rehabilitation there was confusion on the subject resulting from:

- the unclearness of the primary intent and purpose of the evaluation process,
- inconsistencies in the measurement protocols used,
- variations in the measuring devices,
- variations in the number and type of measures used,
- lack of standardization of reporting results,
- ambiguity of the concepts and underlying theories,
- inadequacy of the measurements taken for patients,
- unavailability of normative data for comparative purposes,
- inability to predict return to work or recurrence of injury.

Conceptually, this confusion is thought to be due to the lack of a clear operational definition of what should constitute a performance profile, which machine or device to use, and the lack of standardization. Consequently, terms

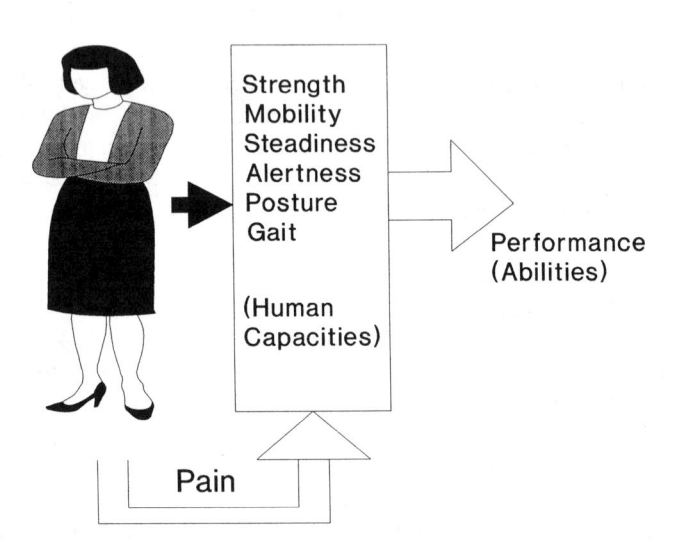

FIGURE 8.1. In the presence of pain or injury, human capacities are modified.

such as "Physical Capacity Evaluation," "Work Capacity Evaluation," "Work Tolerance Screening," "Functional Capacity Assessment," and "Functional Ability Evaluation" were, and still are, being used interchangeably, and in some instances mistakenly. The term functional capacity assessment is generic and is commonly used to describe a variety of assessment techniques (Abdel-Moty, Khalil, Fishbain et al., 1991; Abdel-Moty, Khalil, Sadek et al., 1992). The term refers to an assessment process rather than an evaluation or a screening method. An *assessment* is an investigation of the body function with reference to expected levels (for example, norms or work demands). An *evaluation* is merely a measurement process to find values or amounts describing performance levels without regard to any expected demand. *Screening* is used to separate individuals according to skills, based on interviews and tests. Screening is useful in referring individuals to appropriate treatment, to training programs, or for proper job placement. Figure 8.2 attempts to classify and clarify some of the terms used in an effort to gain consistency in reporting.

The evaluation of human performance depends on measurement. There are some important characteristics that an accurate measuring technique (instrument and methods) should offer (Table 8.1): validity; reliability; sensitivity; lack of redundancy, bias, and contamination; objectivity; comparability; and sophisticated technology. It is absolutely critical that the questions in

Human Performance Terms

Physical Capacities	Functional Capacities	Work Capacities	Cognitive Capacities
Structure and functional limits of the body (physical tolerance limits)	Physical capacities to perform specific job and/or activities of daily living	Structural and functional limits in the work environment (work tolerance level)	Mental faculties
↓	↓	↓	↓
Physical Abilities	Functional Abilities	Work Abilities	Cognitive Abilities
Capacities modified Behavioral, environmental, and physical limitations * (acceptable maximum performance)	Functional capacities modified by behavioral, environmental, and physical limitations (acceptable functional tolerances)	Acceptable functional tolerances in work environment (actual or simulated)	Cognitive capacities modified by behavioral, environmental, and physical limitations

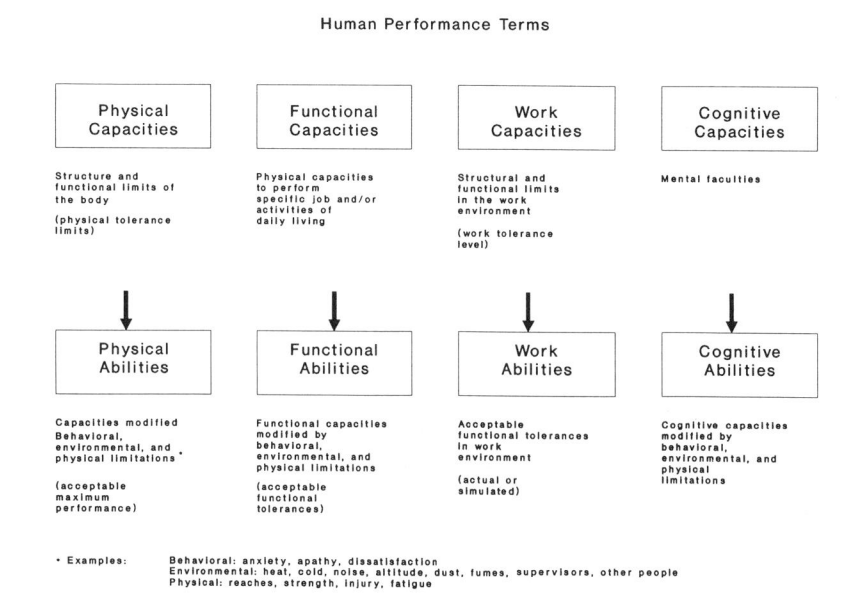

* Examples: Behavioral: anxiety, apathy, dissatisfaction
Environmental: heat, cold, noise, altitude, dust, fumes, supervisors, other people
Physical: reaches, strength, injury, fatigue

FIGURE 8.2. A classification of terms used to describe human performance.

TABLE 8.1   Factors in Performance Assessment

Validity
Does the technique measure what it is intended to measure?
Does it measure other qualities as well?
Can one make useful predictions based on the measurement?
Is the test relevant to the purpose of the measurement?
Do test results correlate with other test scores?
Do they correlate with scores obtained at other points in time?

Reliability
Is the measuring technique consistent?
Is it consistent over time as well as across situations?
Can you get the same results if another evaluator performs the testing?
How much variability should you allow when tests are repeated?

Sensitivity
Is the technique precise enough to detect small, yet significant, differences or changes?
Can the test really separate the highly motivated person from the less motivated person?
Is the measuring technique appropriate for use by healthy as well as injured individuals?

Redundancy
Is the measurement useful and adequate for inclusion in the performance profile?
How appropriate is the technique in providing new information?
Are there measures that are repeated?
How do measures overlap?

Bias
Is the measurement influenced by any factor other than the actual performance of the individual?

Contamination
Was performance influenced by the evaluator's prejudgement of the individual's performance?
Are the instructions clear and void of suggestive wording?

Objectivity
Does the evaluation method provide numerical values?
Is the evaluation based on the evaluator's judgment or patient's display of function?

Comparability
Is there an available set of norms that can be used to determine the relative achievement of the individual in comparison to matched individuals?

Technology
Does the measuring instrument posses enough technological sophistication to allow reproducibility, standardization, and quantification?
Was the test developed specifically for the purpose of evaluating injured individuals?
Was it developed under other circumstances and is being adapted?

Table 8.1 be asked before drawing conclusions using any measuring procedure or device.

Additionally, the following recommendations can be offered (Abdel-Moty, Khalil, Sadek et al., 1992):

1. The measurement process should be labeled accurately to describe whether the objective is to evaluate (or screen, or assess) functional (or physical, or work) abilities (or capacities).

2. Multiple measures should be used. Reliance on single measures (for example, strength) can be misleading.

3. Findings of physical evaluations do not necessarily translate into knowledge of functional or work performance abilities. Nonspecific tests may not reflect the actual demands of repetitive job activities (Rodgers, 1988).

4. Behavioral factors and secondary gain issues should be considered after assessment, so as not to bias the observation. During testing, all behaviors and observations should be documented. Moreover, evaluators should ensure that the subject fully understands instructions and directions.

5. Patients may not exert themselves to a maximum, as pain may inhibit or produce fear when physical exertion is requested. Therefore, performance measures among low back pain patients are the product of both physical and psychological factors.

6. Evaluators should incorporate data from other clinical, behavioral, and vocational assessments in order to establish a comprehensive view of the actual levels of function, as well as factors interfering with performance.

7. Evaluation requires professional skills in designing, performing, and analyzing screening instruments. Reliance on computer-generated reports can be misleading and may have serious consequences.

8. No one evaluation machine is perfect for all patients; no one machine is ideal for all situations; no one machine can assess all aspects of human performance; no one system is foolproof; no one system provides the definitive answer regarding return to work; there is no machine that can provide a composite picture of performance.

9. Evaluation findings should be cautiously interpreted when describing "function," "impairments," "limitations," "restrictions," or "disabilities." *Impairment* refers to "a stable and persisting defect in the individual at the organic level, which stems from known or unknown molecular, cellular, physiological, or structural disorders" (Susser, 1990). Impairment may lead to limitations in function and may decrease the capacity to adapt to the environment (Spektor, 1990). *Limitations*, on the other hand, have been defined as "what the patients cannot do either because of mechanical/physiological problems or because the specified activity causes intolerable pain" (Battista, 1990). *Restrictions* are defined as "what the patient should not do because doing it will either aggravate the condition, delay healing, or possibly constitute a risk to the health" (Battista, 1990). *Disability* refers to a "stable and persisting physical or psychological dysfunction at the personal level, which stems from the limitations imposed by the impairment and by the individual's psychological reaction to it" (Susser, 1990).

10. Evaluation findings should not be interpreted by the evaluator alone. Input from vocational as well as medical experts should be included and correlated.

COMPONENTS OF THE HUMAN PERFORMANCE PROFILE

Measurements of the human performance profile (HPP) can be grouped under four main categories.

1. Physical measures
2. Physiological measures
3. Functional measures
4. Work-related measures

Physical Measures

In this category, evaluation is specific to each individual's *physical* activity, including anthropometric characteristics, strength, posture, flexibility, kinesiology, and psychomotor abilities. These are detailed below in terms of the underlying concepts and the data collection procedures.

Evaluation of Anthropometric Characteristics
Anthropometry (anthropo—human; and metricos—of or pertaining to measurement) is concerned with the physical measurement of people. Anthropometry is a branch of physical anthropology, which in turn is a branch of anthropology. Anthropology is the science of man, including his evolution and characteristics. Physical anthropology deals with physical measurement, both quantitative (length, weights, etc.) and qualitative (for example, color). Anthropometry deals with the quantitative portion of physical anthropology.

Human measurements are essential for designing personal attire (for example, clothes) and for designing equipment (tools, chairs, beds). Workspace dimensions cannot be properly established without knowledge of the dimensions of its occupants. As many as 135 various measures have been taken in some anthropometric surveys. However, the number of measures needed for general design purposes is considerably less, and only a few measures may be needed for specific purposes.

Anthropometric data can be obtained through anthropometric surveys. Anthropometric surveys are made on the same basis as all other statistical surveys. A sample is taken from a certain population, and measurements are taken for the subjects in the sample and projected for the whole population. Population and sample selection depend on the objective of the survey. Data are population specific. Data cannot be taken from one population and used for another without a great deal of rationalization and testing. For example, a survey that is taken using the population of the United States and used to design equipment for American users cannot be directly used to design equipment for the Japanese or Chinese people.

Two types of anthropometric data can be collected: static and dynamic. Static anthropometry (anatomical dimensions of the human body during static postures) deals with simple measurements that include weight, height, length, breadth, width, circumference, and other parameters of body segments. Dynamic (or functional) anthropometry deals with the measurement of the body resulting from movement, such as ranges of joints motion, reaches, and deviations from the neutral position. While static anthropometry is needed for the design of dead space, dynamic anthropometry is needed for workspaces. Both are of prime importance to any task or equipment design.

Linear measurements of body segments can be taken between identifiable landmarks on the human body (Fig. 8.3). Static and dynamic measurements can be obtained in order to accurately describe the individual's space needs. Anthropometric measurements are frequently implemented in the design and analysis of workplaces for the reduction of stresses and improvement of safety (Abdel-Moty and Khalil 1988c, 1988d).

Testing Muscular Strength

Muscular strength has been the primary focus of human performance evaluators in industry and in rehabilitation. Strength testing has been recommended as an integral component of the evaluation of workers. Chaffin (1974), Cady et al. (1979), Keyserling (1982), Keyserling et al. (1980), Biering-Sorensen (1984), Nachemson and Lindh (1969), and others have studied strength as a potential risk factor for back injuries and report that weaker individuals may be more prone to musculoskeletal injuries than stronger individuals. An exception to this position was recently given by Battie et al. (1989). It is, however, a generally accepted concept in ergonomics that stronger people have better tolerance for heavy or sustained task demands.

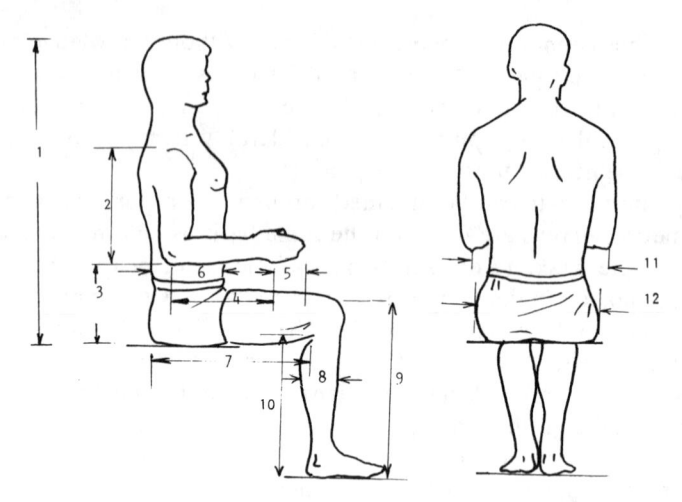

FIGURE 8.3. Many standard static and functional anthropometric dimensions can be used to describe the human body. Examples are: (1) sitting height, (2) upper arm length, (3) elbow height, (4) forearm length, (5) hand length, (6) waist circumference, (7) buttock popliteal length, (8) calf girth, (9) knee height, (10) popliteal height, (11) elbow to elbow width, and (12) hip breadth.

The term *muscle strength* is used to describe the maximal force muscles can exert in a single voluntary effort, that is, the muscular capacity to exert force under prescribed conditions (McCormick and Sanders, 1982). Smidt et al (1983) define strength as the ability of a muscle or muscle group to generate a movement around a body axis or point. The measurement of such force or strength ability depends on several factors including (1) intrinsic muscle strength, (2) subject's motivation and other psychological factors, (3) experimenter's instructions, and (4) measurement index (peak or average values).

Muscular strength is a term often used interchangeably with muscle force. *Muscle force* represents an action of a vector with magnitude and direction acting on an object. Force is defined by mass multiplied by acceleration. For muscles to support or move an external load, it must generate an internal force of such a magnitude that when it is multiplied by the effort arm it produces a torque equal to or greater than the torque produced by the external force of the load multiplied by its lever arm. Muscular force generation is, therefore, a function of the muscle's contractile properties, as well as the external biomechanical system measuring that force.

The power of muscular movement is brought about by the contraction of the muscle fibers. In muscles, contraction is an active shortening of the muscle resulting in a reduction in the distance between its ends. The firing of the embedded motor nerve endings cause the actin and myosin protein fibers of

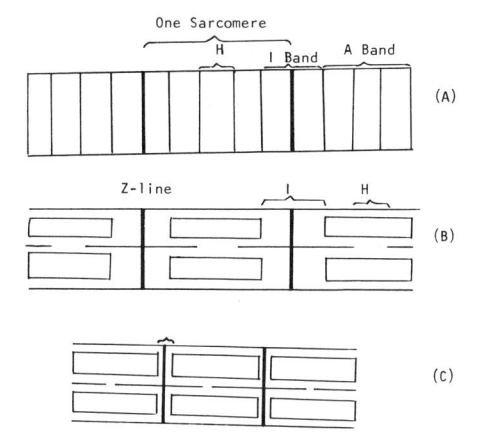

FIGURE 8.4. The unit of the skeletal muscle (sarcomere) showing the striated bands (A). The sarcomere in a relaxed (B) and a contracted (C) condition (actin and myosin filaments slide, bringing the Z line closer).

the muscle to *slide* past each other, bringing the muscle ends closer (Fig. 8.4). Thus, the muscle gets shorter and bulkier. The fibers can contract to approximately 57% of their resting length, which generally controls the distance of movement of the limbs to which the muscle is attached. The amount of muscle contraction depends on the strength and duration of the stimulus, the weight of the load, and the temperature. Continuous contraction encourages the accumulation of metabolites (for example, lactic acid), causing fatigue. Nerve fibers control contraction (Fig. 8.5). The sensory nerves monitor the state of contraction, while the motor nerves deliver the impulses to activate muscle contraction. Muscle fibers contract completely or not at all (ALL or NONE law). This depends on the neural impulse stimulus reaching a threshold value. The muscles intended for more precise movements have less muscle fibers per nerve axon, providing more refined control. The Golgi tendon body and the muscle spindles provide signals to the central nervous system (CNS), which enable the cerebellum to regulate muscle work and to provide tension for posture, equilibrium, and balance. Muscular contraction is brought about by virtue of fiber recruitment. The more the load on the muscle, the more the number of fibers recruited. This is controlled by the CNS and is dependent on the number of fibers in the muscle and the nerve supply to these fibers. The strength of a muscle, at any particular contraction, is therefore a function of the number of nerve impulses its fibers receive at any one unit of time. The contraction process requires a large number of nerve impulses to fire the fibers in unison in order to produce a strong contraction. The number of fibers that are signaled to fire by the CNS is determined from learned clues as to

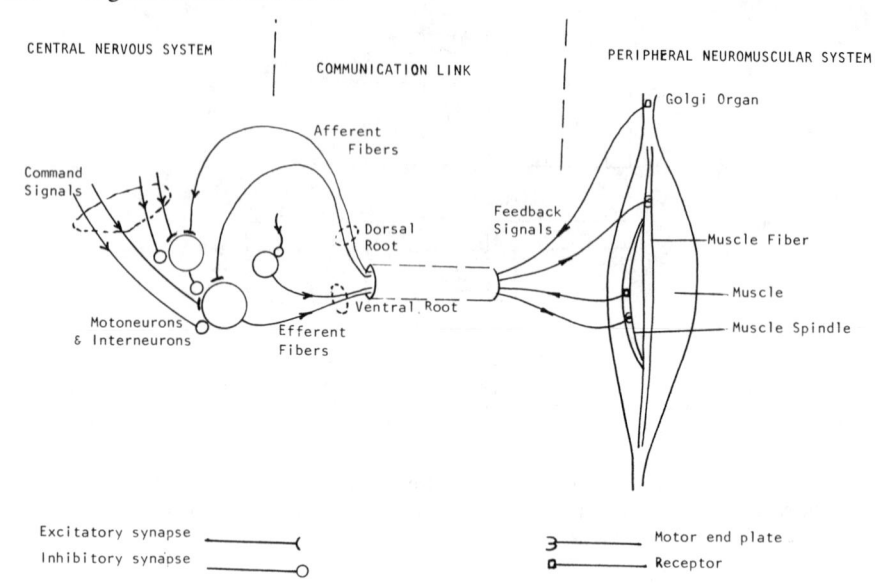

FIGURE 8.5. Schematic diagram of the neromuscular control loop, its pathways, and main components.

the anticipated weight of the item to be moved (Khalil, Waly, Zaki, 1990). After the motion has begun, neuromuscular feedback allows the brain to determine how many more or less firings are needed. As indicated earlier, muscle fibers contract according to the all or none principle; that is, the fibers will either contract fully or they will not contract at all. The more the contraction force needed, the more the number of fibers recruited.

The strength of a muscle can be defined in terms of its resistance to tension, namely, the tension necessary to cause the muscle fibers to slip past each other or break. It is the opposite of the slipping action that causes muscles to contract. Muscular strength varies from muscle to muscle, from individual to individual, and according to a number of parameters that affect muscular performance. The absolute strength of a muscle, all other factors being equal, is roughly proportional to its circumference. Two muscles having the same circumference, however, might vary in strength due to a number of factors. Some of these are as follows:

1. Percentage of fat tissue in the muscle Fat lacks contractile power and limits the rate and extent of the shortening of the muscle fiber.

2. Tissue temperature When the temperature is slightly higher than normal, the muscle viscosity is lowered, the chemical reactions of contraction are increased, and the contraction process is improved. Warm-up exercises increase the temperature and help the state of contraction.

3. Metabolism Foodstuff and oxygen supplying energy to the muscle must be available for the muscle to continue performing.

4. Fatigue Fatigue reduces power, contraction ability, and excitability of muscles. All of these can affect strength.

5. Work Recovery Muscles having good circulation will perform longer, and those with faster recovery rate will be ready to work sooner.

6. Training Muscles can be made stronger by causing them to work against increasing loads.

7. Age Strength increases rapidly in the teens, more slowly in the early 20s, reaches a maximum by the middle to late 20s, remains at this level for 5–10 years, and thereafter declines slowly but continuously. Studies have shown that by age 40 muscle strength in men is approximately 90% of the maximum reached in the late 20s, by age 50 it is about 85%, and by 60 it is about 60% of maximum (Fig. 8.6).

8. Occupation Muscle strength is affected to a great extent by a person's occupation. For example, white collar workers, on the average, are weaker in muscular strength than manual workers.

9. Equipment and Devices These can augment strength. For example, backrests on seats increase pushing strength; footrests increase pulling

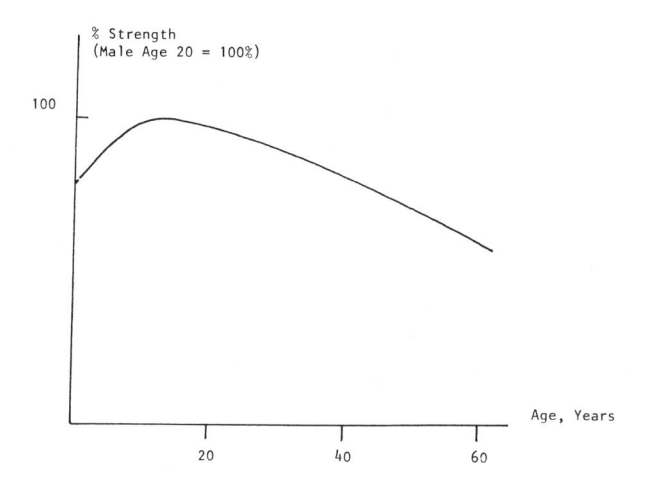

FIGURE 8.6. Isometric strength as a function of age for men.

strength, as do some restraining harnesses and seat belts. By restricting body movement, however, seat belts might also eliminate a more efficient position for muscular effort. Clothing in some cases restricts the range of body movement, deserving consideration in activities requiring muscular strength.

The two main techniques that have been used to assess muscle strength are (1) static strength testing method, and (2) dynamic strength testing methods (restricted or free isoinertial, psychophysical, and isokinetic).

Static Strength Testing
In the static strength testing method, strength is determined by measuring muscular exertion while the body part is restrained against motion. Static testing measures the person's ability to exert isometric muscle strength in a defined posture or several defined postures. The American Industrial Hygiene Association in its Ergonomics Guide for the Assessment of Human Strength has standardized the procedures for the measurement of human static strength (Chaffin, 1975). For healthy individuals, maximum voluntary contraction (MVC) is a commonly used measure of strength. In static testing, the individual is capable of exercising better body control than in dynamic testing. Static testing also affords a better capability of focusing on the output of a defined muscle group or set of muscle groups. Chaffin and Andersson (1984) indicate that the static strength testing method is safe, reliable, and practical for the healthy and able individual. Likewise, Keyserling (1982) indicates that isometric strength testing is an effective and valid tool that can be used by industry as part of an employee selection and training program. Chaffin et al. (1978) and Keyserling et al. (1980) suggest static strength testing as a screening method for reducing occupational back injuries that they believe occur due to a mismatch between the strength of the employee and job demands.

There are, however, drawbacks in utilizing maximum voluntary contraction protocols of static strength testing, usually used for testing of healthy individuals, for the evaluation of muscle strength in injured persons. Hansson et al. (1984) calculates the load on the lumbar spine resulting from the forces imposed by maximum isometric strength testing and conclude that those loads are close to the level of structural failure. These findings suggest that exposing LBP sufferers to *maximum* level of isometric strength testing may induce unnecessary levels of stress on the spine. Mayer, Gatchel, Kishino, Keeley, Capra et al. (1985) eliminate the isometric component from their patients' strength testing protocols due to safety considerations. Protocols for maximum voluntary contraction in static strength measurement may place the typical chronic pain sufferer under risk of further injury during the evaluation. It also does not take into consideration the level at which they would be willing to function consistently in normal life. Moreover, maximum isometric strength testing was not found to predict industrial back pain reports accurately (Battie et al., 1989). For these reasons, Khalil, Goldberg et al. (1987) suggest the use of psychophysical measures of acceptable maximum effort (AME) in static testing of strength ability in low back pain patients, rather than using maximum voluntary contraction (MVC) levels (for more details of the AME Protocol refer to the section on the evaluation of people with chronic pain or injury at the end of this chapter).

In all protocols for static strength testing, subjects assume postures (Fig. 8.7) simulating tasks similar in nature to those encountered in their daily activities and in their work environment (Chaffin, 1975; NIOSH, 1981; Khalil, Goldberg et al., 1987). The selected postures (Fig. 8.8a–h) allow for assessments of the capabilities of the individual's muscular system and can be used for the purpose of evaluating work capacity and for preemployment screening (Chaffin, 1974; Chaffin et al., 1978; Keyserling, 1982; Keyserling et al., 1980).

Static Strength Testing Positions The following static strength testing positions have been used by many researchers and practitioners including the authors and have been proved to be safe and useful in providing information about the strength characteristics of individuals. In testing static strength, the following procedure can be followed:

1. Subject assumes the specified static testing position
2. Subject applies the force in the specified direction

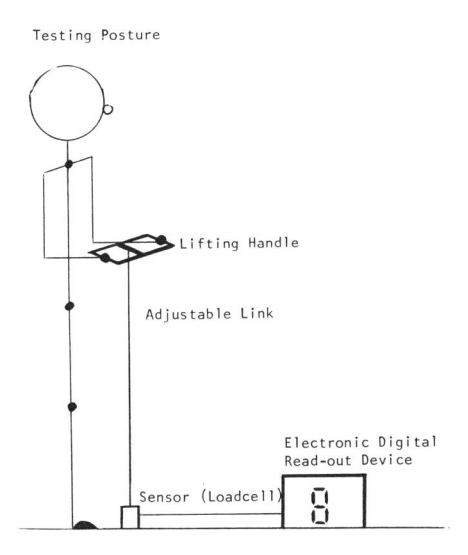

FIGURE 8.7. Basic set-up for the assessment of static strength.

114   Ergonomics in Back Pain

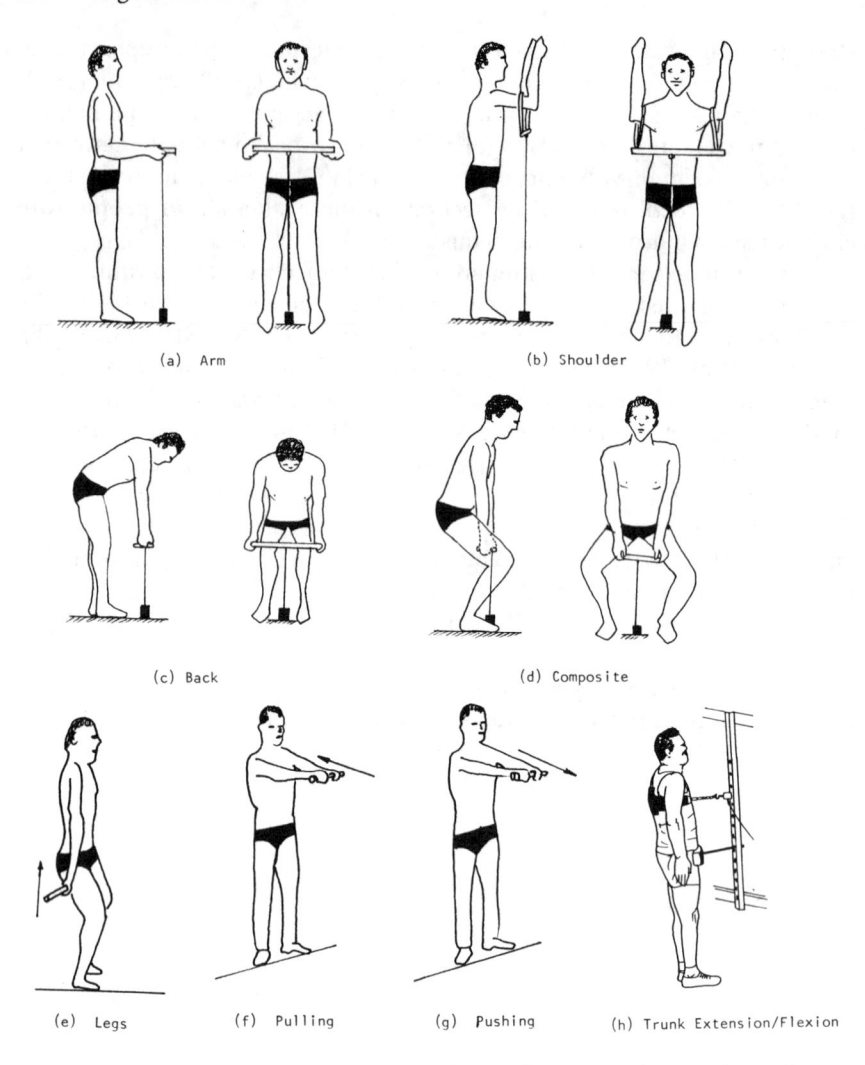

(a) Arm (b) Shoulder

(c) Back (d) Composite

(e) Legs (f) Pulling (g) Pushing (h) Trunk Extension/Flexion

FIGURE 8.8. Schematic illustration of the various testing postures for assessing static strength abilities.

3. Subject builds up his/her muscle tension slowly without any jerks, twists, or disruptive motions
4. When the subject reaches maximum voluntary contraction level (for healthy subjects), or the point beyond which he/she perceives discomfort and pain level becomes unacceptable (for patients with low back injury), he/she holds that level of tension for a four-second count

Principles and Methods of Interventions   115

5. During the four-second period, the average and maximum forces give a value of MVC or AME (depending on the instructions given) for the first repetition in the specific testing position
6. Subject repeats the MVC or AME measurement three times for the given position

Evaluation of Grip Strength. Grip strength is assessed by requesting individuals to grasp a handle connected to an electronic dynamometer and apply force while the elbow is kept at 90° flexion. Subjects are instructed to squeeze as much as they can while exhaling. Three attempts are performed for each hand, starting with the right hand. The grip strength value reported is the average of the peak value obtained for the three attempts.

Arm Strength Testing Position. The functional objective of this measure is to determine the individual's ability to support objects with the forearm and hand at 90° flexion at the elbow, with the upper arm hanging to the sides. This posture (Fig. 8.8a) simulates the task of supporting food trays, boxes, books, babies, etc. Many tasks in our daily lives and in the workplace require this type of posture both while standing and sitting.

Shoulder Strength Testing Position. The functional objective of this measure is to determine the individual's ability to lift objects overhead (Fig. 8.8b). Many situations dictated by the environment require lifting overhead, such as putting plates in a kitchen cabinet or placing a bag on a high shelf.

Back Strength Testing Position. The functional objective of this test is to determine the individual's ability to lift bulky objects or to lift when a bent-knee technique is not feasible. This posture (Fig. 8.8c) is commonly used by many people, although it may stress the back. Many designs or situations of the work environment dictate this type of lift. Examples are getting a suitcase out of the trunk of a car, reaching to pick up a frozen food package from an open-type freezer in a supermarket, reaching to get a container from a back row of a shelf, lifting a baby from a crib, or attempting to lift a large-size object that does not fit between the legs. All these situations require back lifting. Some people, in fact, cannot perform any other type of lifting because of knee injuries, balance problems, arthritis, etc.

Composite Strength Testing Position. The functional objective of this measure is to determine the individual's ability to lift objects in a semisqaut position, which is more commonly known as leg lifting. The measurement in this posture (Fig. 8.8d) reflects both the back and leg strength. The posture is generally recommended for lifting objects. It relies on the strength of the leg muscles to perform the lifting, rather than the relatively weaker back muscles. It is convenient for infrequent lifting of small objects that can fit between the legs. It represents an initial posture for lifting objects.

Leg Strength Testing Position. The functional objective of this measure is to determine the individual's leg muscle strength. This posture (Fig. 8.8e) is used for lifting some objects using the leg muscles while keeping the back straight, with pronated hands hanging to the sides of the body. An example of this is lifting a stretcher, lifting the edge of a table, etc.

Pushing Strength Testing Position. Approximately 20% of overexertion injuries have been associated with pushing and pulling acts (NIOSH, 1981). The objective of this measure is to determine the individual's pushing abilities. This posture (Fig. 8.8f) is used to push furniture, close/open heavy doors, slide boxes on the floor or on a surface, or push a grocery cart in a supermarket. Foot slip potential is very high while performing pushing and pulling acts (Pope et al., 1984). This variable should therefore be controlled by using platform surfaces with similar friction before comparing pushing strength results. Variations in test locations can produce variations in results obtained, therefore, specifying the exact posture while pushing is important.

Pulling Strength Testing Position. The functional objective of this measure is to determine the individual's ability to pull objects toward the body while standing up. This posture (Fig. 8.8g) is encountered in many daily activities such as opening/closing doors, pulling boxes off a conveyer belt, opening file cabinets. Specifying the exact posture and foot location is important if pulling results are to be compared.

Trunk Flexion/Extension Strength Testing Position. Quantification of trunk and abdominal muscle strength provides one component of a battery of tests for measurement of functional capacities or abilities. Quantification of functional abilities (and the change in these abilities after treatment starts) as well as the measurement of trunk muscles' capacity in LBP patients, have been done repeatedly (Asfour et al. 1990, Khalil, Asfour, Waly et al., 1987a, b, Mayer, Smith et al., 1985; Alston et al., 1966; Mellin, 1989). Nachemson and Lindh (1969) found no clear relationship between trunk muscle strength and the incidence of LBP. The ratio between flexion and extension strength has been found to be of no prognostic value of future occurrence of LBP (Biering-Sorensen, 1984). Many authors report decreased trunk muscle strength in LBP patients (for example, Asfour et al. 1990, Khalil, Asfour, Waly et al., 1987a, b, Mayer, Smith et al., 1985). Trunk extension and flexion strengths were found to be associated with LBP and progress due to treatment, but extension had stronger correlation (Mellin, 1989). For measuring trunk flexion/extension, the posture depicted in Figure 8.7h can be used. In this test the subject stands erect and the pelvis is stabilized against a special frame. A belt is placed around the torso of the subject and is attached to a fixed-length chain linked to a force-measuring device. The subject is asked to apply a pulling force against the belt by performing back extension. The acceptable maximum effort concept for measuring strength can also be used for this purpose.

Dynamic Strength Testing
When muscular exertion results in body-segment motion, the resulting force measured is referred to as dynamic strength. This is more complicated than the static strength measurement method. Since this method requires body motion, muscular force is required to accelerate body mass, and this in turn assists the muscle in producing additional force output (Chaffin and Andersson, 1984). Predicting a person's dynamic strength ability has been attempted by many researchers (Park and Chaffin, 1974; Pytel and Kamon, 1981; Asfour et al., 1984; Khalil et al., 1984; Khalil, Waly et al., 1987; Chaffin and Andersson, 1984; Emmanuel et al., 1956; Snook et al., 1970; Ayoub et al., 1978). Results from dynamic strength testing are thought to be better predictors of functional strength capacities. Caution should be exercised when dynamic protocols are used to test patients. Dynamic strength testing techniques may not be suitable for application in some back injury cases. Back pain sufferers run a higher risk of further injury and exacerbation of symptoms during dynamic strength testing than during static testing. This is because they have less control over the external weight moved and on their body's movement abilities.

One example of measuring strength dynamically is through the use of isokinetic testing protocols. The term isokinetic implies a constant speed. Isokinetic testing measures muscle strength capability while body segments move at a constant speed. The measurement of isokinetic strength requires a high degree of technological instrumentation. There are many commercial systems available for such assessment. The differences in the design and mechanical characteristics between these systems can, potentially, alter the values of force or torque measured. This makes direct comparison between results of various studies difficult. Caution should be exercised when attempting to extrapolate test data from one machine to the other (Thompson et al., 1989).

Evaluation of Static Posture
For the evaluation of static posture, a posture chart can be used as shown in Figure 8.9. The subject is asked to stand behind the posture chart, facing away from the evaluator. Posture is scored relative to deviations from the horizon-

Good   Fair   Poor

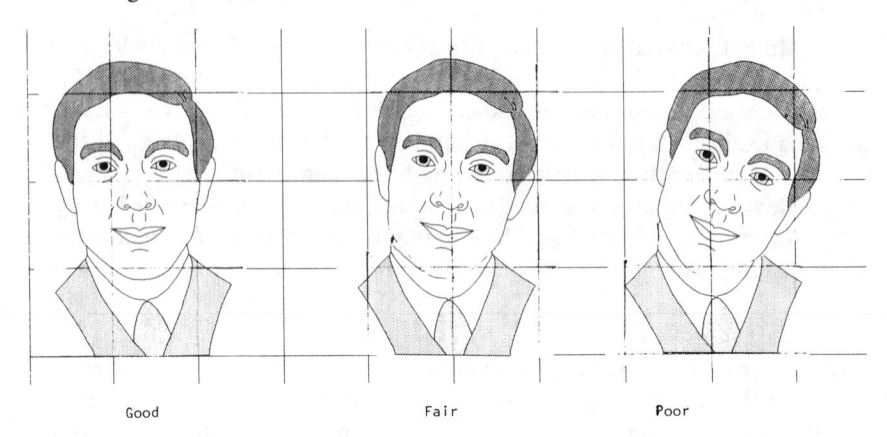

FIGURE 8.9. For the evaluation of posture, charts can be used where the horizontal and vertical alignment of various body segments (the head in this case) are checked. A score is then given in terms of the deviation from a center line. The procedure is repeated for the shoulders, spine, hips, ankles, upper and lower back, trunk, and abdomen. When applicable, lateral and back views should be obtained. Commerical posture charts are available for this purpose.

tal and vertical lines of the chart, with specific reference to the alignment of the iliac crest and lumbar curves. The patient is then asked to turn and stand with his/her shoulder touching the mid-line of the chart, and deviations are once again scored. A total score is provided as a percentage deviation from normal. During this evaluation, videographic recordings can be conducted in order to document posture alignment for further computerized analysis. Proper posture is an essential ingredient in the prevention of health problems, particularly LBP.

Evaluation of Flexibility
Many investigators have documented decreased spinal flexibility among low back pain patients before treatment and have reported significant improvement due to rehabilitation (Khalil, Asfour et al., 1992, 1986; Mayer and Gatchel, 1988, Mayer et al., 1984). Others have found that lateral flexion and rotation correlated significantly with back disability and progress in rehabilitation (Mellin, 1989). Measures of hip mobility were also found to correlate with pain (Rosomoff, et al. 1989; Mellin, 1989; Fairbank et al., 1984). Measuring the range of motion of different body segments is a very important component in the determination of physical function/disability and in the evaluation of treatment and rehabilitation programs. Assessment of joint motion and musculoskeletal function can vary from a simple visual estimation to a three-dimensional analysis of body motions. There are several commercially available devices that can be used for measuring body

(A) Gravity Goniometer

(B) Fluid Goniometer

(C) Universal Goniometer

(D) Electronic/Digital Goniometers

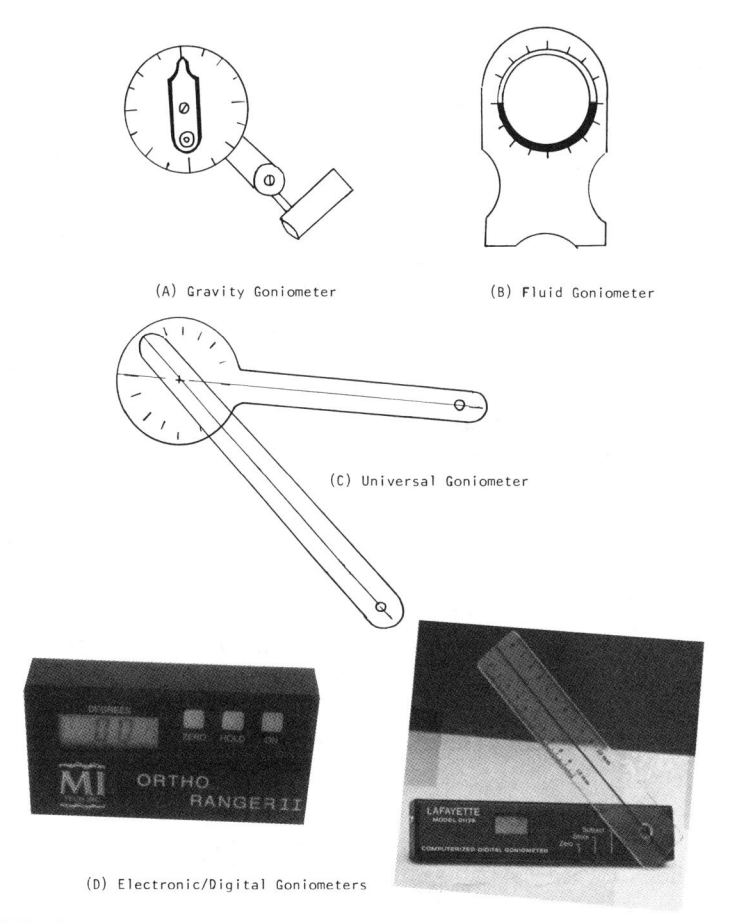

FIGURE 8.10. Examples of flexibility measuring tools.

segments' ranges of motion (Fig 8.10). Using the simple universal goniometer is the most popular method to assess ranges of motion of joints. The popularity of the universal goniometric technique has been primarily attributed to its versatility, ease of use, and low cost.

The reliability of universal goniometric measurements has been a topic of considerable concern. Some studies report high reliability, and others report low reliability (Rothstein et al., 1983; Fish and Wingate, 1985; Petherick et al., 1988). Reliability of the goniometric measurements appears to depend on a variety of factors including

- joint measured,
- goniometer placement,

- patient characteristics,
- experience of the examiner, and
- nature of the patient's problem.

The introduction of new devices, such as electronic inclinometers, are intended to increase the accuracy and the reliability of goniometric measurements. The Orthoranger, an electronic inclinometer, was introduced by Orthotronics Inc., M.I. Technologies. The device was reported to be reliable in measuring active range of motion (ROM) (Clapper and Wolf, 1988). The Orthoranger II™, by MI Tech Inc. (Daytona Beach, FL), is smaller in size; it is easier to use; the transducer is contained in one box with the processing unit. The reliability and accuracy of this device were confirmed by Pisciotta (1987) and by bench testing conducted by the authors. Another type of electronic inclinometer was introduced by Cybex. It incorporates several electronic processing features. A newer, more sophisticated range of motion assessment system (ROMAS) was introduced by Verimed, Inc. (Fort Lauderdale, FL). One of the advantages of using electronic inclinometers over traditional goniometers is measurement precision. It was observed in clinical trials that angles measured by electronic inclinometers are reported in one degree increments, while those measured by the universal goniometer are reported in five degree increments (Zaki et al., 1992). The AMA has published its most recent guidelines, which are based on using one or more inclinometers to measure complex movements of the body.

Kinesiological Evaluation
Several kinesiological measurements can be made. Some of the pertinent ones include forward walking speed, sway (forward, backward, and lateral), balance, and weight distribution under the feet.

Evaluation of Walking Speed
Walking speed could be used as an additional index of functional abilities. One simple measurement can be obtained by requesting the subject to walk forward for a known distance (for example, 15 feet) as fast as possible. The time (t) spent to walk this distance (x) is recorded digitally. The walking speed is calculated by dividing the distance (x) by the time (t) and reporting results in units of feet per second.

Evaluation of Postural Sway, Weight
Distribution and Balance
Evaluation of postural sway can be performed by using specialized biomechanical performance analysis systems such as the Ariel System™. The patient is asked to stand on a force platform. The shift of the body's center

of pressure is recorded for a selected period of time (Fig. 8.11). The same record is used to determine weight distribution under the feet. For the evaluation of balance, the patient is asked to assume a certain stance (for example, one legged, tandem, or stepped) for a defined period of time and the amount of sway is quantified. This can be reported as linear displacement of the body center of gravity in one direction (x or y). A more sensitive measure of sway has been found to be the area of sway defined by x × y (Khalil, Abdel-Moty, Sadek et al., 1992).

Evaluation of Psychomotor Abilities
Low back pain patients were found to have slower reaction time than individuals of equivalent age (Abdel-Moty, Khalil, Asfour, Howard, et al.,

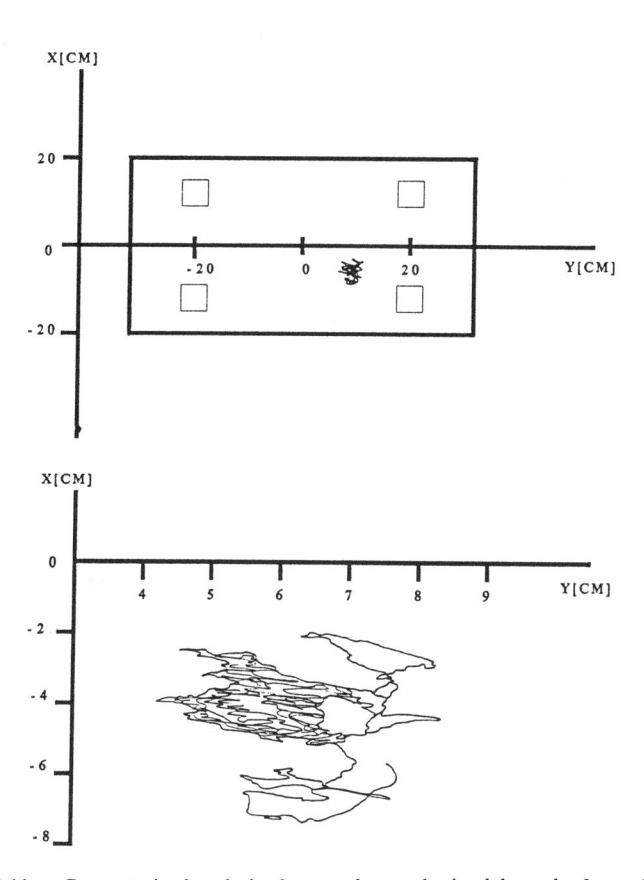

FIGURE 8.11. Computerized analysis of postural sway obtained through a force platform and the Ariel Performance Analysis System. The area of sway is enlarged in the X and Y direction, then measured. Norms need to be established for sway measuring systems and for the population.

1989). Moreover, reaction times were found to improve with pain reduction, successful rehabilitation, and restoration of functional capacities. Some of the measures of reaction time include upper and/or lower extremity reaction time. Reaction time is the time taken from the onset of a signal (stimulus) to the initiation of a response. Reaction time measurement can be made by using any standard reaction time testing machines (for example, Lafayette Reaction Time Apparatus™, Fig. 8.12). Reaction time is measured by the time lapse between the onset of a stimulus (sound and light) and the patient response to the stimulus (pressing a button). Typically, a series of trials are made, and an average reaction time score across trials is reported.

Hand steadiness can be measured by requesting the patient to place a metal stylus into a hole of given size for a period of time (for example, 15 seconds) without touching the sides (Fig. 8.13). Each time the needle touches the metal edge of the hole, an impulse counter records the number of touches. While holding the needle in the hole, the patient is not permitted to support his/her elbow. Analysis is made of the total number of touches to get an index of hand steadiness.

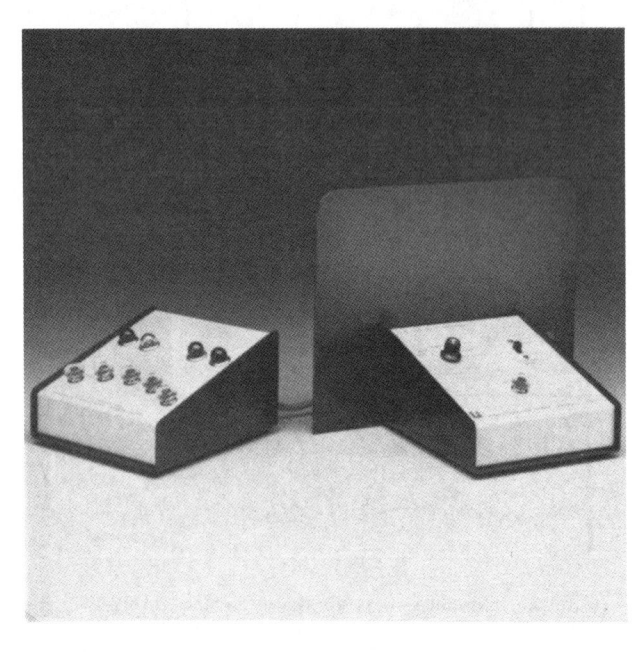

FIGURE 8.12. Apparatus for measuring reaction time.

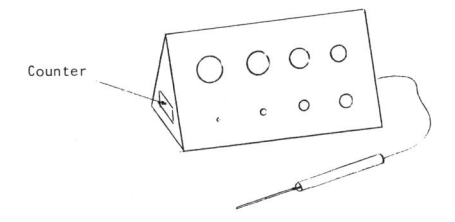

FIGURE 8.13. Apparatus for measuring hand steadiness.

Physiological Measures

The human activities of moving, exerting forces, and doing work require a certain amount of energy to be supplied to the body's systems and to the muscles that perform these functions. The two basic components necessary for the supply of human energy are food and oxygen. The changes that foodstuff and oxygen are subjected to are known as *metabolism,* a chemical process in which foodstuff is converted into energy in the form of mechanical work and heat (Fig. 8.14). When energy is produced in the absence of oxygen, the process is known as *anaerobic metabolism*. In presence of oxygen, this process is known as *aerobic metabolism*. The human body is capable of producing energy aerobically as well as anaerobically, however, the later process cannot be continued for a long period of time.

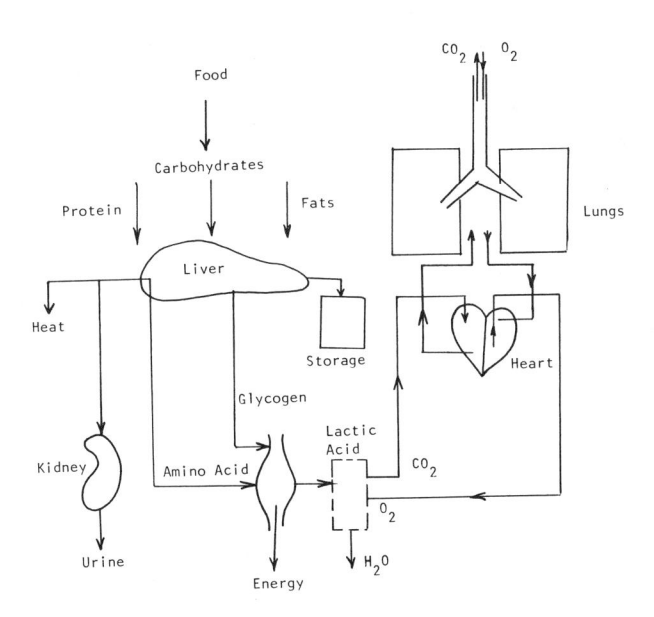

FIGURE 8.14. A schematic diagram illustrating the process of the production of energy from food and oxygen.

Up to 75% of the energy required by the body comes from carbohydrates. Glucose is the simplest form of carbohydrates. It is the form in which carbohydrates are transmitted in the blood, and it constitutes an immediate energy source. Fats are absorbed and stored in deposits in the body. They can be used on recall and broken down the same way as carbohydrates, after they have passed through the liver. Protein is directly involved in tissue maintenance, enzyme formation, and as a source of energy. As previously mentioned, energy can be liberated with or without the existence of oxygen. In case of oxygen absence, the reaction cannot continue because of the formation of lactic acid in the muscles. Moreover, aerobic energy output is much higher than anaerobic energy output. (Glucose can provide 20 times more energy per mole aerobically than anaerobically.) This should make it clear that the existence of oxygen is the major factor for continued, efficient energy release.

Food sources are controlled by human diet, and oxygen supply is controlled by the cardiovascular and respiratory systems. Oxygen is inhaled with air and passes to the lungs, where an exchange of oxygen and carbon dioxide in the venous blood occurs. Blood corpuscles saturated with oxygen are passed from the left atrium to the left ventricle, where it is pumped in arteries to the rest of the body. Venous blood saturated with carbon dioxide is returned from the body through veins to the right atrium. It is then passed to the right ventricle, where it is pumped to the lungs and the cycle is repeated.

The larger demand for oxygen needed for work is met by speeding up the mechanisms controlling its supply, such as the respiration rate and the heart rate. The rate of metabolism can be measured by direct measurement of the heat liberated as a result of the biochemical reaction or by indirect measurement, such as oxygen consumption rate.

The analogy between the function of the human machine and the automobile, a human-made machine, is very interesting. In order for a car to run on idle, it requires a certain amount of fuel and air. If it is to start moving, more fuel and air are required. Similarly, in the human machine a certain amount of food and oxygen is required to keep a person idling (sustain life). If he/she is to work, more food and more oxygen will be needed.

In human terms, a certain amount of energy is needed to keep humans alive and maintain their bodies in an inactive state. This amount of energy is provided through basal metabolism. Basal metabolism is the rate of energy expenditure in the complete absence of voluntary muscular activity. This rate is at its lowest when a person is asleep. It is advantageous to distinguish between that rate and the resting metabolic rate, which is generally the baseline for most working situations. In the latter a person is not engaged in an activity, but he/she could be maintaining a posture such as sitting or standing. In such instances, metabolic rate is higher than the basal rate. The resting metabolic rate requirement (cost) is stable. Metabolic cost increases with the increase of activity. Oxygen uptake and other physiological parameters increase. When work stress is removed all physiological parameters tend to go back to their basal value (complete recovery). The period of time needed for this adjustment is known as the recovery period.

Sufficient oxygen supply to the muscle in needed to oxidize the lactic acid formed as a result of the work activity. If this supply is not adequate during the work period, the muscle will not stop functioning immediately, it will develop an *oxygen debt* (Fig. 8.15). This oxygen debt is equivalent to the quantity required by the contracting muscles over and above the quantity actually supplied to them during their activity. This quantity has to be paid back after work performance. This amount of oxygen is not borrowed from another source as the term might indicate; rather, it is a delayed payment for work that was produced anaerobically.

The oxygen requirement varies with work load. A basal oxygen consumption rate is about 0.25 liters/minute. Light or moderate tasks require about three times the basal quantity, and heavy work requirements are about eight times. For an untrained person, the maximum rate at which oxygen can be consumed is about 8–12 times the basal rate of consumption. This quantity could be increased to 20 times with training. When moderate or heavy work is performed, glycogen or glucose is used to build up high energy phosphate bonds to supply energy for muscular contraction. It is clear that if the oxygen demand is greater than that supplied by the cardiovascular system, lactic acid builds up and oxygen debt is developed. The development of lactic acid causes a decline in muscle action until it finally stops. It may be useful to know an individual's oxygen debt tolerance. This may allow a prediction of his performance. For an untrained person, the maximum tolerable debt is about ten liters. If the difference between oxygen required and oxygen uptake can be reduced, an individual can sustain long periods of activities. A long

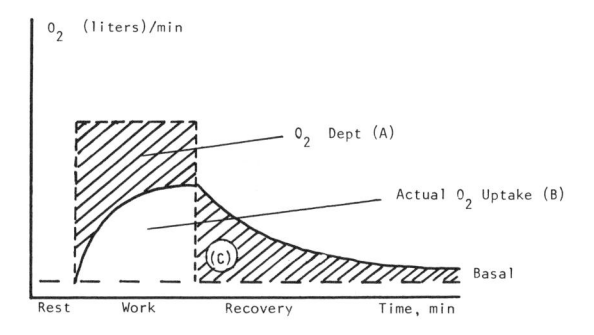

FIGURE 8.15. Rest–work recovery cycle showing the oxygen debt (A + B = B + C).

distance runner must have a high oxygen uptake (liter/min). In short distance running, it is impossible to increase oxygen uptake in such a short time, and oxygen has to be paid back during the recovery period.

Rate of oxygen uptake depends on supply of oxygen and exchange of oxygen. Supply is controlled by both the ventilation rate and blood circulation. Deep breathing increases the partial pressure of oxygen in the alveolar air. More oxygen can then be picked up by the blood. This is due to the fact that the rate of passage of oxygen into blood is determined by pressure of the gas in the alveoli rather than by its percentage. The capacity of blood to carry oxygen is based on the hemoglobin content of the blood. The more hemoglobin in the blood, the greater its capacity for carrying oxygen. Unloading of oxygen at the tissues is increased by physical activity to a value between 2 and 2.5 its original value. Limits on long strenuous work can be predicted based on an individual's capacity for oxygen uptake during work and the body's capacity for oxygen debt. For example, if the oxygen cost (that is, the oxygen rate requirement for a task) and the oxygen debt are known, a prediction of performance can be obtained. This is done by comparing the oxygen rate requirement (cost) with what the individual can supply through aerobic and anaerobic means:

$$\text{Oxygen Cost} < \frac{\text{Rate of Oxygen Uptake} \times \text{Duration of Task} + \text{Oxygen Debt}}{\text{Duration of Task}}$$

If the oxygen cost of the task is less than what the individual is capable of supplying, the task will be within the individual's physiological capacities. If a person has an oxygen uptake capacity of x liters/min, his/her oxygen debt capacity is y liters/min, and a task requires z liters/min, then he/she can perform this task for a period of p minutes where:

$$p = \frac{y}{(z - x)}$$

Such predictions can be made for workers as well as athletes.

Evaluation of Cardiopulmonary Capacity

Pulmonary capacity can be assessed using a submaximal stress test to predict maximum oxygen uptake (VO_2max) (Astrand, 1976). Prior to testing, the subjects should be screened for potential contraindications to exercise participation (American College of Sports Medicine, 1976). The test can be performed on a motorized treadmill using the Balke Protocol (Balke, 1971). This protocol uses smaller transitional work loads throughout the test. Subjects are connected to a standard 12-lead electrocardiography machine. They perform fast-walking on the treadmill at a constant speed of three miles per hour, with an increase in tread grade occurring every minute until they attain 85% of their age-adjusted maximal heart rate. Maximal oxygen uptake (VO$_2$max) is predicted using the Astrand-Rhyming Monogram (Astrand, 1960), corrected for the subject's age. This method requires the subjects to have attained an exercise heart rate greater than 120 beats per minute during their treadmill stress test, with prediction of functional capacity based on the gender of the subject, the highest attainable treadmill work load (either symptom-limited or 85% of their age-adjusted maximal heart rate), and the measured heart rate of the subject at the completion of their highest attainable work load. Should symptoms limit the exercise capacity of the subject before they reach their target heart rate (American College of Sports Medicine, 1976), the work load at the highest symptom-limited work load and corresponding pulse rate is used to predict VO$_2$max.

Human Work

Work can be physical or mental. Only physical work will be discussed. The term human work is vague and requires clarification. *Work*, as defined in physics, is a force acting through distance. It obeys the following law:

$$\text{Work Done} = \text{Force Applied} \times \text{Distance Moved}$$

Thus, for example, moving an object a distance of 3 feet by applying a force of 5 pounds throughout this distance is equivalent to 15 foot-pounds of work. However, a person supporting a load, or pushing against a fixed object is not performing *work*, as so defined; yet he is still expending energy. The latter type of work is merely a function of force and time, and not a function of force and distance. It should, therefore, not be confused with the term work as classically defined. Since both types require muscular activity, it has been suggested that the term *effort* be used instead of work (Kroemer, 1970). The first type of human work can be referred to as dynamic effort, and the second type as static effort. The term work should only be used in dynamic situations and is measured in units of mechanical work (for example, foot-pounds).

Classification of Human Effort

The terms work, effort, contraction, action, exercise, train, and load have been used rather loosely to describe human/musculoskeletal activities. All of these terms refer to internal effort of the muscle as modified by the characteristics of the external load imposed on the muscle in a specified human posture or movement pattern. It is important to properly define terms when reporting strength information and describing human activities. Failure to do so can result in misinterpretation of information.

Static Activities These are activities where muscle effort is expended in a static posture. In this category human effort is a function of force and time (not displacement). There are two terms used to describe effort in static activities: static effort and isometric effort.

Static Effort This term is sometimes referred to as static work, even though it is not work in the classic sense. Static effort creates muscular contraction, which in turn creates physical pressure within muscle tissue. Prolonged and constant pressure restricts blood circulation to the muscle. Since there is only minimal oxygen supply to the muscles, this condition creates a rapid development of oxygen debt and muscle fatigue. Consequently, whenever possible, static loading of muscles should be avoided. Examples of static loading include prolonged fixed sitting postures and lifting then holding or carrying for long distances. Muscle effort expended in static activities could be at a submaximal level, as in the case of holding a light weight, or could be maximal, as in the condition of maximum voluntary contraction (MVC) in static postures.

Isometric Effort This term is sometimes referred to as isometric work and refers only to the internal effort within the muscle. The term isometric implies that muscle length remains constant during tension without regard to the amount of tension. Since no *visible* motion occurs during isometric effort, the term isometric sometimes is used interchangeably with the term static. It is preferred to use the term isometric effort when describing muscle action and the term static effort when describing task related activities.

Dynamic Activities Dynamic activity (work) is characterized by intermittent contractions and relaxations of muscles. During the contraction, blood circulation is restricted in a way similar to that of static effort. However, during the phases of relaxation, circulation and oxygen supply is much higher than during muscle contraction. It follows, therefore, that the performance of dynamic work permits muscles to have better oxygen balance, with a lessened rate of development of muscle fatigue. Dynamic activities take on many forms: isotonic, isokinetic, isoinertial, positive and negative, and eccentric and concentric efforts.

Isotonic Effort The term isotonic effort refers only to the internal effort of the muscle. The term isotonic implies a constant tension (force) of the muscle without specifying its length. This term is sometimes used when a constant load is being moved through a distance. In the latter condition, the use of the term is inaccurate since the tension (force) developed by the muscle changes with changing length and changing mechanical advantage.

Isokinetic Effort The term isokinetic implies a constant speed with variable resistance that accommodates to the muscle's ability to generate force. In isokinetic work the muscle changes its length at the same rate throughout the range of motion. The term is used to indicate the situation where a constant velocity in the muscle is maintained even if the muscle changes its length. As the muscle length changes, the resistance alters in a manner that keeps the velocity constant. This permits maintenance of the same dynamic load throughout contraction.

Isoinertial Effort This term is used to indicate constant external load throughout the range of motion. Two types of isoinertial effort can be identified: unrestricted isoinertial effort (free) and restricted isoinertial work. Unrestricted refers to the fact that speed and trajectory of movement are not externally controlled. An example of such activity is lifting a box. The term restricted isoinertial work is used to indicate constant external load throughout the range of motion. Restricted refers to the fact that the trajectory of movement is limited by the design of the task. An example of this type of activity is using a Universal™ weight training machine or a Liftest machine for determining dynamic lifting capacity (Kroemer, 1983).

Positive and Negative Effort Human effort can also be classified as positive or negative. *Positive effort* is done when the muscle shortens. An example of this is lifting a load. *Negative effort* is done when the muscle elongates. An example of this would be lowering a load. Since both types of effort involve the movement of a certain load through a distance (that is, work), their mechanical work value will be equal, but their physiological cost will be different. The energy expended in positive effort is more than that used for negative effort. Therefore, whenever possible, design the workplace to make use of this fact. An example of this would be to use drop deliveries instead of carrying objects to a fixed location.

Concentric and Eccentric Effort *Concentric effort* is a dynamic effort in which muscle length decreases (that is, muscle responsible for movement becomes shorter); in other words, the origin and insertion are drawn together. For example, the biceps contracts concentrically when raising weight. *Eccentric effort* is a dynamic effort in which muscle length increases while effort is still being exerted; in other words, the origin and insertion are drawn apart. This is a case in which resisting external force which usually exceeds the force generated by the muscle. If the external force does not exceed the muscle force, isometric effort will occur.

Fatigue

Fatigue is a sense of weariness due to labor or exertion. Within this broad definition, the term fatigue describes various conditions that can result in such a sense of weariness. A subjective sensation of fatigue is the most common form exhibited. A feeling of tiredness prevails. This feeling will persist as long as its cause is present. It may increase with time until it reaches a certain limit, after which breakdown occurs. A change in the physiological functions of the human body is usually associated with the state of fatigue. Some physiological changes such as heart rate, oxygen consumption, and muscular activity can be directly monitored as measures of fatigue. Work performance is heavily affected by fatigue. A fatigued human being exhibits a diminished capacity for doing work. His/her judgment may be impaired and productivity decreased. The most common type of fatigue is muscular fatigue. This is characterized by a decreased capacity for exerting force and by greater time needed for muscular movement. Muscular fatigue is caused essentially by the build-up of lactic acid, a waste product, which tends to restrict continued activity of the muscle. Fatigued muscles lose some of their ability to maintain contractile power. Mental fatigue is characterized by decreased capacity for thinking, rationalizing, and judgment. It is usually caused by prolonged periods of mental activity and/or excessive mental stress. Psychological fatigue is characterized by psychologically induced inability to function, tension, sleepiness, and headaches. It is caused by severe continuous daily fatigue. It can develop into a state of chronic fatigue where the symptoms of physical or mental fatigue are exhibited even in the absence of physical or mental stress.

Fatigue can be avoided by removing its cause and providing periods for recovery. In physical fatigue the most effective cure is rest. The greater the stress, the greater the risk of fatigue, the longer the rest period should be. Hence, work/rest scheduling becomes a critical factor is avoiding fatigue.

Endurance
Endurance is the ability to maintain an activity over a period of time. It is a function of the total energy cost of the activity and the energy expended. There are certain human variables that determine endurance, such as age, sex, and body build. Two terms describing endurance conditions are used interchangeably: muscular and cardiovascular endurance. *Muscular endurance* is the ability of muscles to continue work. Muscular endurance is related to the magnitude of force. People can maintain maximum effort very briefly, whereas they can maintain a force of approximately 25% or less of their own maximum for ten minutes or more (McCormick and Sanders, 1982). Muscular endurance is the opposite of muscular fatigue. *Cardiovascular endurance* is the ability of the cardio-pulmonary system to continue meeting the demands of the body for energy to sustain work.

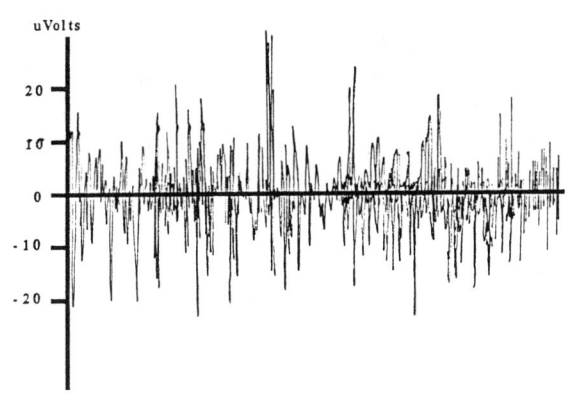

FIGURE 8.16. EMG recording from the biceps muscle during maximum voluntary contraction (MVC).

Electromyography

The process of recording, displaying, and accurately presenting the electrical activity of an active muscle is referred to as electromyography (EMG). It is the technique of mapping an electro-chemical-mechanical phenomena taking place in the neuromuscular system when muscles contract. There are two types of electromyographic recording techniques: (1) through the use of transcutaneous surface electrodes, and (2) through needle or wire electrodes inserted into the muscle. While surface recording produces gross presentation of the contracting muscle (Fig. 8.16), needle electrodes pick up signals from a more specific area of the muscle or are capable of detecting discharges from a single motor unit (Fig. 8.17). In surface EMG there are many external factors that can affect the quality and, subsequently, the information carried by the EMG signals. Among these factors are the type of recording instrument (electrodes, amplifiers, filters, etc.), length of leads, interelectrode distance, electrode ori-

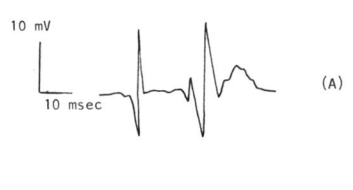

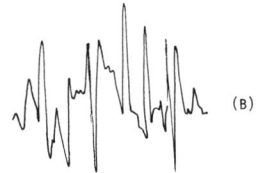

FIGURE 8.17. Sample EMG recording showing two (A) and a number of (B) superimposed action potentials (interference pattern).

entation and configuration, skin preparation and temperature, movement artifacts, and interference from other electrical equipment, and electrical grounding. A primary advantage of using surface electrodes is that they are noninvasive and can be easily applied with virtually no discomfort.

Assuming adequate control of all external factors, the resulting EMG activity is usually a rather complex signal. In order to describe, statistically, the information contained in this waveform, proper processing techniques should be used. Existing computer capabilities are being widely used in designing automated EMG analysis systems (Khalil, 1973; Moty and Khalil, 1986; Basmajian et al., 1975; Bergmans, 1973; Grieve and Cavanah, 1973; Gerber et al., 1984; Hausmanowa-Petrusevicz and Kopec, 1983; Jackson, 1982; Khalil, Asfour, Waly, 1988, Kopec et al., 1973; Rose and Willison, 1967; Basmajian and Deluca, 1985). The basic requirement in these automated systems is their ability to measure the amplitude and frequency characteristics of the EMG signals accurately and comprehensively.

Electromyographic Processing Techniques
Techniques for processing the digitized electromyography (EMG) can be based on a variety of amplitude and frequency measures (Table 8.2 and 8.3). Figure 8.18 displays the process of EMG analysis.

TABLE 8.2 Amplitude Measures

Mean Rectified (MR)
Full Wave Rectified Integral (FWRI)
Root Mean Square (RMS) Value
Sum of Voltage Excursions (SVE)
Range of Amplitudes (RA)
Amplitudes Standard Deviation (SD) and Variance (V)
Entropy (H) and Redundancy (D)
Mean, Mode, Median
Amplitude density function (Histogram)

TABLE 8.3 Frequency Measures

Average Zero Crossings (AZC)
Inter Spikes Interval (ISI) histogram
Frequency profile or power spectrum
Average firing rate
Median frequency
Mean frequency
Band width

Principles and Methods of Interventions 133

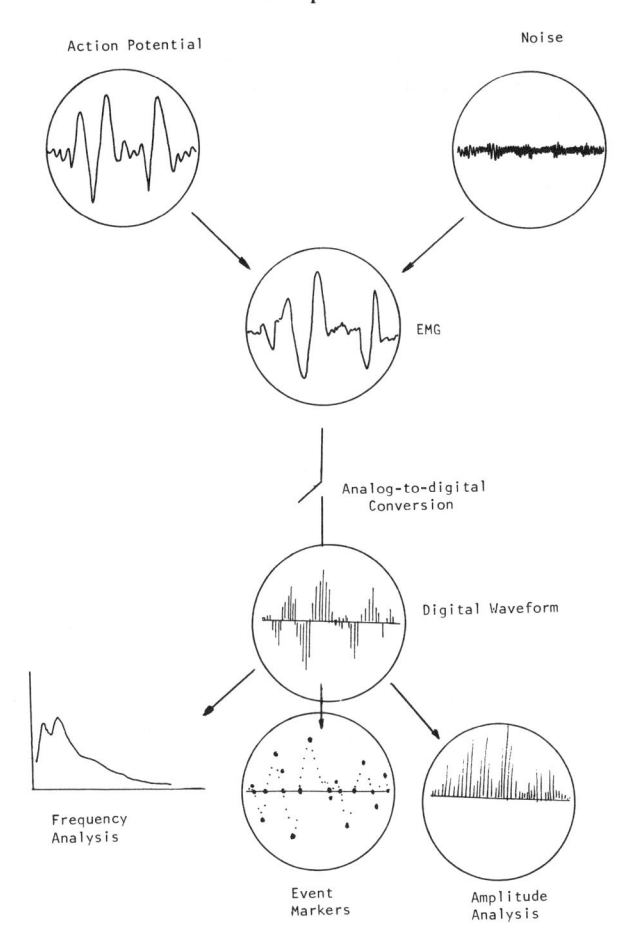

FIGURE 8.18. The process of EMG analysis where the EMG signal (action potential and noise) is filtered, digitized, and analyzed in order to obtain information describing the amplitude and frequency contents of the signal (Moty and Khalil, 1987).

Amplitude Analysis This type of analysis results in the development of indices that describe the magnitude of the signal.

Measures of signal amplitude have been correlated with physiological entities such as muscle strength, muscle fatigue, rate of motor units firing, and synchronization (Abdel-Moty, Khalil, Rosomoff, and Rosomoff, 1987; Basmajian and DeLuca, 1985; Bigland-Ritchie, 1981). (Synchronization is the effect of two or more motor units discharging during the same time interval.) Most of these studies agree that there is a relationship between EMG amplitude and muscle force (Khalil 1973). The Mean Rectified, Full

Wave Rectified Integral, and Root Mean Square values are used to measure the amplitude of the motor units action potentials (Basmajian and DeLuca, 1985). The RMS measure defines the average value of the rectified signal. The FWRI value reflects the energy or power in the signal over an arbitrary period of time. By integrating the EMG waveform, the intensity of muscular activity is measured. The sum of voltage excursions (SVE) is the summation of the absolute amplitudes that exceed an arbitrary threshold (for example, 35 uV).

Even though amplitude analysis is of more interest in rehabilitation, it involves difficulties as to equipment calibration and signal amplification. This constitutes a major problem not only in comparing results of different studies, but also in interpreting results based on the use of amplitude measures only.

Frequency Analysis Frequency domain analysis proved to be as valuable and sometimes superior to the time domain one (Berzuini et al., 1982). This type of analysis involves extensive calculation and requires computer-based approaches. Frequency analysis breaks the complex signal into basic components occurring in preselected frequency bands.

The power spectrum of the signal (Fig. 8.19) describes the distribution of the average power of the signal in the frequency domain. The spectrum of the EMG signal is characterized by the existence of one peak and multiple firing rate peaks. The parameters that have been identified as affecting the presence of the firing peaks are the firing of the individual motor units and the degree of synchronization (Agarwal, 1975; Sato, 1982; Lago and Jones, 1977). The mean and median frequency parameters are considered to be the

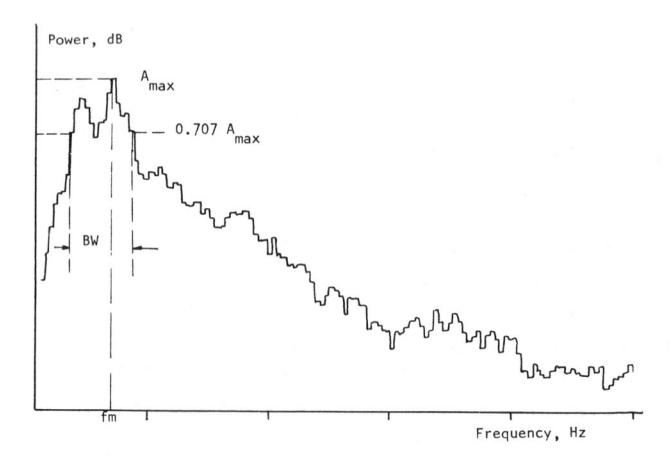

FIGURE 8.19. Example of the frequency spectrum of the EMG showing the band width (BW) and the mode frequency (Fm).

most reliable (Basmajian and DeLuca, 1985). It is possible to draw conclusions of physiological interest from spectral analysis. For example, it was found that the high frequency activity diminished and the low frequency activity increased during fatiguing muscle contractions, presumably due to decrease in muscle fiber propagation velocity (Kaiser and Petersen, 1965). The median frequency of the spectrum was also shown to be a consistent estimator of the conduction velocity and to be more reliable and less sensitive to noise than other estimators (Stulen and Deluca, 1981; Sadoyama et al., 1983). Kranz and associates (1983) find that the median frequency drops progressively during muscle contraction. Lindstrom (1975) reports that the force in a muscle fiber is proportional to the average discharge frequency. Basmajian and DeLuca (1985) show that the amplitude of the power density spectrum increases with the action potentials of motor units that have been additionally recruited. In addition, they show that the spectral characteristics are also affected by the synchronization of the motor units.

The parameter of frequency could also be defined in terms of the number of zero crossings and the number of peaks (turning points) in the waveform (Fig. 8.18). The number of zero crossings per unit time was found to be proportional to the conduction velocity (Inbar and Noujaim, 1984; Hagg, 1981). The average firing rate may be estimated from knowledge of the zero-crossing rate.

Electromyographic recording and analysis can be useful in many areas with respect to evaluation, treatment, and research in rehabilitation. Among these are

- studying the neuromuscular system's response to treatment modalities;
- describing muscle activity and its characteristics at a certain point in time;
- assessing work-related stresses—such as the effect of posture, workplace design, equipment design, or mechanical vibration—on muscular performance and fatigue-related factors;
- rationalizing body mechanics principles to prevent injury and reduce stress;
- validating biomechanical models.

Utilization of the EMG in a variety of applications in rehabilitation requires the availability of EMG processing. There are several EMG systems available that have varying degrees of capability, purpose, and expense. These systems can be classified as follows:

1. Software packages that can be used in conjunction with a computer and an amplifier to analyze the EMG signals for research applications (Moty and Khalil, 1987; Abdel-Moty, Khalil, Rosomoff, and Rosomoff, 1988).

2. Small portable EMG units that can be used in biofeedback applications (Fishbain et al., 1989)
3. Advanced systems for single site and bilateral recording that can be used for biofeedback and muscle reeducation applications (Asfour et al., 1990; Khalil, Asfour, Waly, et al., 1987b; Abdel-Moty, Diaz et al., 1992).
4. Sophisticated and complicated clinical systems that can be used in multiple site recording and for clinical assessment of muscular physiology especially with respect to needle EMG

In several intervention strategies, rehabilitation engineers and therapists might find it useful to use the less sophisticated systems, provided they possess sufficient accuracy and reliability. For research applications, a computerized automated system for quantitative EMG processing is needed to evaluate the functional capacities of the neuromuscular system in many aspects. For muscle reeducation and biofeedback purposes, package systems of less technological sophistication are usually adequate. In Chapter 11 of this book several cases were selected for presentation to illustrate a variety of clinical situations where computerized EMG was used to augment standard medical techniques as a diagnostic and/or evaluation tool.

Functional Measures

It is important to evaluate low back pain (LBP) patients' abilities to perform activities of daily living. Several measures can be taken. The more pertinent ones are

- sitting tolerance (minutes),
- standing tolerance (minutes),
- walking tolerance (distance and time),
- squatting and kneeling (number),
- stair climbing (number of steps or flights),
- manual handling abilities (lifting, carrying, pushing, and pulling).

Evaluation of Tolerances
Patients' tolerances in the categories of sitting, standing, walking, squatting, kneeling, and climbing are evaluated through direct observation and measurement of the patient's performance and behavior.

To evaluate sitting tolerance, the patient may be requested to sit in a *regular* chair. Posture should be standardized: with elbows supported and feet flat on a stool or a footrest. The patient may be allowed to perform productive activity while sitting. Frequency of postural changes is recorded, as well as patient's self-report of change in discomfort.

Standing tolerance can be measured by having the patient assume a comfortable standing posture while alternating feet on a footstool.

The patient's walking tolerance is measured by the time elapsed and the distance traveled (or number of laps). In doing walking activity, pacing should be emphasized.

Squatting and kneeling abilities are measured after demonstrating to the patient the proper manner of performing these activities. Squatting should be performed with the support of a railing and with emphasis on maintaining proper posture and proper body mechanics. Number of squats (whether full or semi) is recorded together with the degree of difficulty in performing the task. Knee precautions should not be ignored when performing this type of activity, as well as in evaluating kneeling ability. Kneeling is measured as the number of times a patient is able to kneel: on one knee and on both knees.

Climbing stairs is measured as the number of steps (or flights) a patient is able to climb and descend continuously. Arms may be used on the rails. In general, all of these activities should be evaluated following the proper instructions and demonstration to the patient.

Evaluation of Weight-Handling Abilities

The techniques currently used for the evaluation of lifting abilities are based on isometric, isokinetic, or isoinertial measurements. Isometric and isokinetic testing protocol can only be used as indicators of muscle strength in performing the lifting activities. Isometric and isokinetic maneuvers do not directly relate to the ability to perform actual lifting activities. Isoinertial evaluation can be performed either using the Liftest approach (Kroemer, 1983) or the psychophysical measurements (Snook et al., 1970; Snook and Ciriello, 1974). Isoinertial testing protocols establish the maximum acceptable levels of performance. In dynamic protocols, the objective is to determine the amount of weight that a person can lift. The Liftest uses a modified weight machine to find the dynamic-load lifting ability. In the psychophysical approach, load is lifted freely in a box. The individual adjusts the weight lifted to reach the maximum amount they are willing to handle manually for a period of time. This load is referred to as the maximum acceptable weight or MAW. Each technique has its merits and drawbacks. Psychophysical testing duplicates the true dynamic nature of lifting tasks in an unrestricted manner. Isokinetic testing, using many of the commercially available machines, is not very realistic since the human body does not move at a constant speed, a condition dictated by isokinetic machines. The isoinertial Liftest confines the trajectory of body movement to the measuring machine. Once again, this is not a natural way of lifting an object in real life situations.

The dynamic test, which allows the determination of maximum lifting capacity, is known as the maximum dynamic weight (MDW) test. In this test, load is added incrementally to the standard size box until the individual is no longer capable of lifting the box (Khalil, Waly et al., 1987). In order to determine dynamic lifting abilities of low back pain patients, the concept of maximum acceptable weight (MAW) of lift seems to be the most justifiable (Khalil, Waly et al., 1987). Maximum acceptable weight is based on a psychophysical dynamic technique suggested by Snook et al. (1967, 1970, 1974) for the determination of lifting abilities in healthy individuals. Subjects are asked to adjust the amount of load in a box (38 × 38 × 25 cm with cut-out handles) to the level they could lift for an extended period of time. The lifting tasks are performed in the saggital plane as follows (Fig. 8.20):

1. lift the box from the floor to 76 cm above the floor with knees bent and back straight (floor to table height)
2. lift the box from 76 cm to 127 cm above the floor (table to shoulder height)
3. lift the box from 127 cm to 175 cm above the floor (shoulder to overhead or reach height)

Each subject can adjust the amount of load lifted until the MAW is reached. Subjects perform the tasks at a certain frequency (repetition rate). A similar protocol can be used with some LBP patients who are capable of performing this type of lifting task. For LBP patients a frequency of one or two lifts per minute may be appropriate for this test. An example of the instructions to the patient for lifting evaluation can be found in Snook et al. (1970, 1974).

Work-Related Measures

The prediction of realistic work behavior and vocational potential requires accurate and oriented assessment of not only physical function, but also psychological and social factors, work tolerances, habits, interpersonal qualities and a host of other factors. In this category, task assessments are performed. The term work evaluation is frequently used to describe this type of assessment. *Work evaluation* is defined as a comprehensive process that

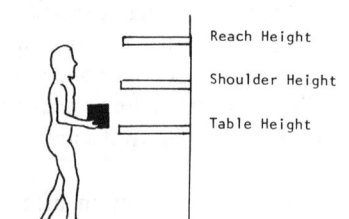

FIGURE 8.20. Dynamic strength testing heights (Khalil, Waly et al., 1987).

systematically uses work, real or simulated, as the focal point for vocational assessment (Esser, 1983). The objective of work evaluation is to help evaluators, as well as workers, realize their highest level of functional independence. The Commission on Accreditation of Rehabilitation Facilities (CARF) provides a list of factors described in the traditional vocational evaluation model. They include physical and psychomotor capacities; intellectual capacities; emotional stability; interests, attitudes, and knowledge; personal, social, and work history; aptitudes; achievements; work skills; work habits; work-related capabilities; job-seeking skills; effects of task performance on symptoms; and many more.

The U.S. Department of Labor (1977, 1981) identifies 20 physical factors essential for matching workers to their job demands. These physical demands express both the physical requirements of the job and the physical capacities (traits) a worker must have to meet job demands. The 20 factors are strength, standing, walking, sitting, lifting, carrying, pushing, pulling, climbing, balancing, stooping, kneeling, crouching, crawling, reaching, handling, fingering, feeling, talking, hearing, and seeing. These factors constitute the basic elements of the work capacity profile.

The evaluation in this category should be goal-oriented; that is, it should evaluate the patient's ability to perform *specific* job-related activities. Two types of evaluation can be performed.

1. **One-time evaluation** with the purpose of evaluating the patient's ability/inability to perform the tasks in single attempts
2. **Full-day assessment** in order to evaluate the patient's work tolerances (ability to perform job tasks for a full work day)

In either case, the objective is to identify and describe work activities that a patient can perform safely and the level of performance in each activity. The knowledge obtained from the evaluation of physical, physiological, and functional abilities can be integrated with work evaluations in order to produce an accurate presentation of a patient's capabilities and limitations. Assessment should be specific to each task and may include simulation of job tasks and evaluation of performance in the simulated environment. Holmes (1985) recommends the use of critical physical demands, those that are more likely to induce onset of symptoms and limit work tolerances.

In this category, patients perform activities similar to those encountered on the job or in activities of daily living in actual or simulated environments. Patients are observed for cooperation, proper use of body mechanics, time required to complete each task, achievement level in each activity, consistency, as well as self-reports of ease and comfort in performance (Abdel-Moty, Khalil, Fishbain et al., 1990; Abdel-Moty, Khalil, Sadek et al., 1990).

Activities of lifting, carrying, pushing, and pulling are simulated with emphasis on object size and shape, handle size and shape, height, weight, and arm/hand carrying positions similar to those used on the job. In addition, in the design of a full-day assessment, the evaluator should consider how often a task is performed on the job. The Department of Labor's classification of job demand characteristics (continuous, frequent, occasional, never) should be used for this purpose. The operational definitions of this type of characterization is given in Appendix E.

EVALUATION OF PEOPLE WITH CHRONIC PAIN OR INJURY

The effects of chronic pain and injury on human performance can be evaluated either by asking the patients about their perception of how much they can or cannot do or by objectively measuring the patients' abilities or limitations. It is recognized that there may be a discrepancy between these two different types of measures (Khalil, Goldberg et al., 1987). As a matter of fact, self-reported measures obtained through questionnaires have been found to correlate poorly with therapist's observations, with spouses' ratings of patients' ability to perform the same activities, and even with patients' self-reports in an interview.

Self-Reported Measures

Health care professionals, in general, rely on patients' self-reports of pain location and level, medication intake, and functional deficiencies in activities of daily living to supplement their clinical evaluations. Patients' ratings of their ability to perform activities have been referred to as *perceived self-efficacy* (Council et al., 1988; Bandura, 1977). When considered in relation to pain, self-efficacy expectancies have typically been defined as a person's perceived ability to cope with pain (Council et al., 1988). In general, patients expectancies of physical impairment and pain have been reported to bear a substantial relationship to actual performance (Council et al., 1988).

The accuracy and validity of self-assessment instruments have been subjected to much scrutiny, especially when comparing a patient's self-assessment of their activity level with a therapist's paper-and-pencil and observational assessments. Discrepancies have been reported in what patients report as their activity level in a self-administered instrument and what they report when interviewed (Spiegel, Hirshfield and Spiegel, 1985; McGinnis et al., 1986). Patients reported requiring more assistance with self-care activities in a self-administered questionnaire than they did in an interview, and appeared more willing to admit difficulties with self-care activities in a self-administered questionnaire than in a personal interview (Spiegel et al., 1985). The difference between what patients report as their functional level and what they can actually do has also been studied (Council et al., 1988; Sanders, 1980).

These discrepancies have been attributed to the possibility that (Spiegel et al., 1985; McGinnis et al., 1986)

- patients may be less willing to admit difficulties to a therapist whom they are meeting for the first time, than they are to report them in a questionnaire;
- patients may be embarrassed to admit having difficulty;
- patients may try to please the interviewer by claiming less difficulty than is actually present;
- patients are anxious;
- patients assume the sick role;
- therapists are trying to demonstrate effectiveness of the rehabilitation program;
- patients and therapists have different interpretations of functional ability;
- patients and therapists use different comparison rules in evaluating functional ability.

Despite the apparent problem with self-reported measures, this type of assessment has been used as an integral component of clinical evaluation. In recent years investigators have developed elaborate functional classification systems designed to evaluate the effects of therapy or rehabilitation on patients' outcomes (Jette, 1980b). Most of these instruments use a four- or five-point multiple-choice scale that orders respondents' degree of dependence in performing several global activities of daily living (Granger and Greer, 1976; Katz et al., 1970). Most studies have reported discrepancies between what patients report as their activity level, on one hand, and what they can actually do based on observations, monitoring, or ratings by spouses. Recent studies indicate that patients as well as healthy individuals underestimate their abilities to perform certain activities of daily living (Abdel-Moty, 1992).

Another dimension of the issue of self-report of activity levels is the lack of information regarding whether the general population of healthy subjects can accurately estimate their abilities to perform daily activities. The absence of such information in the available literature makes it statistically unsupportable to conclude that patients' reports of abilities are inaccurate. Additionally, while some studies report inconsistencies between self-report and observations, others tend to disagree.

Self-reported measures are an important tool for health care professionals. They can be used to complement the therapist's interview, thus enhancing the therapist's awareness of existing problems with self-care (Spiegel, Hirshfield and Spiegel, 1985). Although patients may report being capable of performing certain tasks, the therapist should know whether or not activities are actually being performed. Self-report questionnaires can also provide information about everyday activities that may be difficult to measure in a rehabilitation setting or under observation. They have been shown to be feasible in quantifying levels of function (Jette, 1980b).

Self-reports are easier to obtain than observations and other measurements. They may be convenient; are less costly; require minimal professional time (McGinnis et al., 1986), address sensitive issues that may be difficult to bring up in a face-to-face interview; and they elicit responses regarding behaviors, knowledge, and attitudes, which are attributes unmeasurable using other devices (Rintala and Willems, 1991). Self-report instruments are, however, of limited usefulness for patients with cognitive impairment or mental handicap (Barnes and Benjamin, 1987). But self-report instruments may be useful in designing treatment approaches in goal-oriented rehabilitation programs. In this case, the patient's self-report of his/her activities of daily living requirements is used to determine the goals of treatment. Therefore inaccuracy in the self-report could result in patients either underachieving or placing unrealistic goals. Self-report instruments have also been used to measure changes upon treatment and have not demonstrated an ability to detect subtle changes in function (Jette, 1980b).

Patients' self-reports have also been suggested as a tool in the evaluation of a rehabilitation program's efficiency and service (McGinnis et al., 1986). The premise that a person's self-statements and appraisal of events, feelings, and behaviors has been considered central to the cognitive-behavioral approach to the management of chronic pain (Kores et al., 1990). Bandura (1986) suggests that performance of actions necessary for meeting treatment goals may be affected by people's judgment of their skills. The author adds that perceived self-efficacy for coping with pain may determine the ways in which people deal with situations associated with pain. This type of self-efficacy expectancies has been found to correlate significantly with tolerance for physical activities (Dolce et al., 1986). Council et al.'s findings (1988) suggest that self-efficacy expectancies ultimately determine performance. Kirsch (1986) argues that self-efficacy ratings reflect behavioral intentions.

Performance Assessment in Rehabilitation

Evaluating functional capacities of an individual is an important undertaking in rehabilitation, work placement, and in screening of individuals with pain. Many agencies, rehabilitation institutes, medical centers, and work programs have developed testing protocols and batteries of tests for various purposes. There are important issues in the evaluation of injured individuals that have to be considered in the development of any battery of tests.

1. A battery of tests is needed for the assessment of functional capacities. The studies that have used single measures (for example, strength tests, Battie et al., 1989), to predict future industrial chronic low back pain have not provided definitive results. This is due to the fact that these studies are based on a limited set of assumptions. For example, it may be assumed that improper lifting is the cause of low back injury. However, as was shown in Chapter 2, lifting represents only 25% of low back injuries, whereas slips and falls result in about 40% of the injuries (Khalil, Asfour, Moty, 1984, 1985). Therefore, concentrating on the assessment of lifting traits alone, such as strength capabilities, without considering other important factors, such as environment for example, may not be adequate.

2. Measures of functional capacities, especially muscle strength, are dependent on many factors, such as age, height, weight, and gender. Therefore, response variables (measures of functional capacity) should be related to the individual characteristics.

3. In order to measure capacities, will individuals with CLBP exert maximum effort? They may not, as pain can inhibit or produce fear when physical exertion is requested. Therefore, functional measures among CLBP patients are the product of both physical and psychological factors. Willingness to exert oneself to a given level of performance is one of possibly several psychological variables that can affect outcome. Indeed, this psychological factor could play a significant role in the level of effort that the patient will demonstrate on the job or in activities of daily living outside the testing environment. As such, the *acceptable* functional levels achieved should be accurate indicators of the maximum level of voluntary effort that the person would be willing to produce outside the test position. This psychophysical concept is called AME, acceptable maximum effort (Khalil, Goldberg et al., 1987).

The Concept of Acceptable Maximum Effort

For the most part, quantification of functional strength among low back pain individuals has been viewed by evaluators as merely a direct extension of strength evaluations for healthy, unimpaired individuals. In general, muscular strength has been assessed through the use of maximum effort protocols, mostly concentrating on a few muscle groups. This has limited the scope of the evaluation and made it difficult to generalize these results to overall task performance. The psychophysical measure of acceptable maximum effort (AME) presented by Khalil, Goldberg et al. (1987) identifies the acceptable levels of strength performance, specifically in patients with chronic LBP. For evaluating strength in persons with chronic pain, AME refers to the maximum level of voluntary effort the person can achieve without an intolerable level of pain or discomfort. It defines the highest functional level that can be attained within the bounds of acceptable pain (Figs. 8.21, 8.22).

In more than 1,200 chronic back pain patients, the AME procedure proved to be safe, reliable, and sensitive to pain perception. It correlates well with physical status when measurement is made at any point during rehabilitation. This psychophysical measure of strength takes into account not only the patient's physical capabilities, but his/her perception of how much they can perform within the boundaries of pain perception. Our work to date in the assessment of functional abilities of patients suffering from LBP indicates that the AME measurement is successful in distinguishing patients in terms of their levels of functional abilities. It is also useful in quantifying the degree to which functional abilities have been restored as a result of rehabilitation (Fig. 8.23). When used relative to strength performance of healthy uninjured individuals of the same age and work group, a functional restoration index (FRI) can be obtained. By definition, the FRI index (AME of pain patients divided by the 50th percentile MVC value of healthy workers) is less than unity for patients prior to rehabilitation and approaches or exceeds unity following successful rehabilitation.

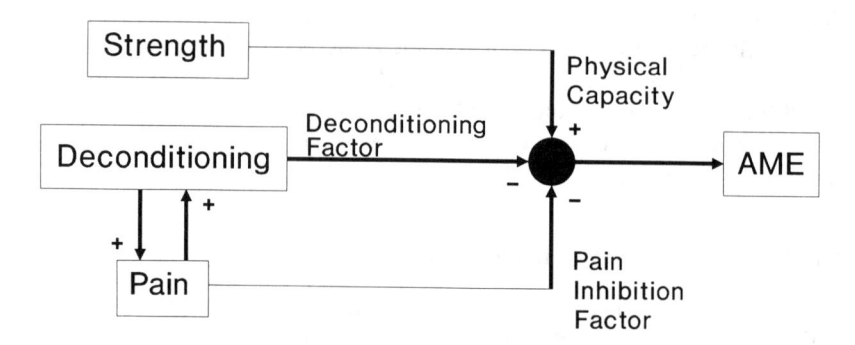

FIGURE 8.21. The AME model: performance Ability (AME) is the result of physical capacity (strength) modified by deconditioning and pain factors.

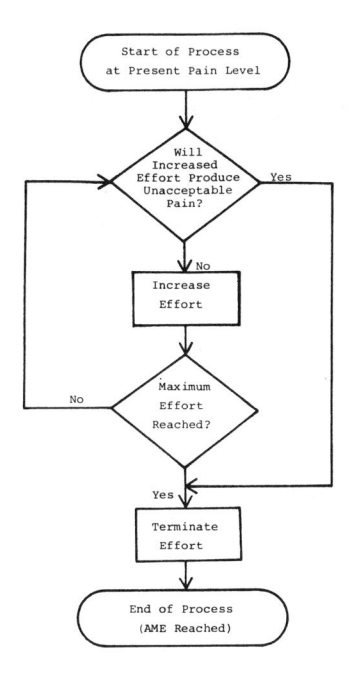

FIGURE 8.22. A flowchart describing the AME test process. (Adopted from Khalil, Goldberg et al, 1987.)

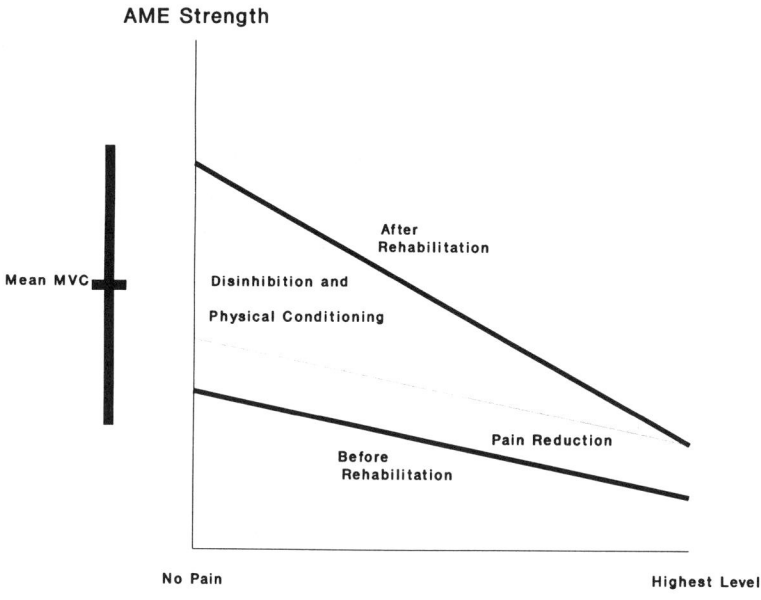

FIGURE 8.23. Conceptually, and as proven from actual testing on patients, AME approximates MVC norms at no-pain condition. As pain increases AME decreases. Following rehabilitation, the same relationship remains. Improvement in AME following rehabilitation may be attributed to pain reduction, disinhibition, and/or physical conditioning.

An Example of Instructions to the Patient When Using the Acceptable Maximum Effort Procedure

If the AME concept is used to test static strength, then standard postures and devices used for static strength measurement can be used (Chaffin, 1975). The testing instructions, however, will be different. An example of instructions follows.

"You are about to be evaluated for overall body strength. You will be requested to assume each of these positions (evaluator points to pictures of the testing positions mounted on the wall) during the assessment. These positions simulate different daily activities such as carrying a tray, putting an object into a kitchen cabinet, lifting an object from the floor, or placing a bag on a high shelf. I will instruct you on how to assume the test positions. While performing the strength tests there is something very important we want you to keep in mind. We know you have pain or discomfort. When I ask you to begin, I want you to build up your strength slowly against the handles of the testing device without any jerks, twists, or disruptive motions. Remember, do not hold your breath at any time. Continue to build your effort until you reach a point at which you believe that any additional increase in effort would cause an intolerable increase in pain or discomfort. You will be asked to hold that level of effort for a slow count of four. How you release the load is very important. Release the load gradually. You will be given a short rest period, and we will repeat the procedure until three values are recorded for each testing position."

It should be noted that the psychophysical AME concept extends beyond static strength testing protocols. It is applicable to dynamic strength testing, as well as to ranges of motion measurement.

9
Principles and Methods of Interventions Through Biofeedback, Muscle Reeducation, and Functional Electric Stimulation

When injury occurs, several physiological and psychological processes are triggered. Musculoskeletal injuries can result in a variety of problems, such as muscular weakness, contractures, pain, reflex inhibition, atrophy, reduced ranges of motion, and many more changes in the structure and function of the musculoskeletal system. Several intervention strategies and methods can be used to alleviate one or all of these problems. Some of these methods are described here.

BIOFEEDBACK

Biofeedback (BF) is the procedure by which information regarding biological activity (for example, muscle contraction, breathing rate, heart rate, etc.) is gathered, processed, and conveyed back to the person (or patient), so that biological activity can be modified under voluntary control (Fig. 9.1). Thus, BF combines learning (by the patient), experience (of the therapist), and technology (the machinery) in order to accomplish treatment goals. Feedback can be provided in two modes: visual and auditory. Methods of feedback fall under several categories including temperature feedback, electromyographic (EMG) feedback, electroencephalographic feedback, and electro-

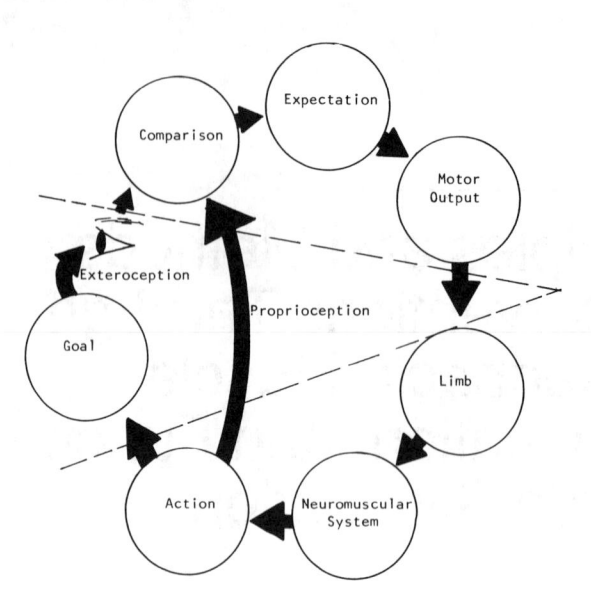

FIGURE 9.1. Basic elements of the feedback loop.

dermal feedback. The most commonly used methods of biofeedback are the temperature and EMG modes.

Temperature Feedback

The principle underlying the use of temperature feedback is that skin temperature is a function of blood flow and blood vessel dilation or constriction, and consequently the state of the sympathetic portion of the autonomic nervous system. Warmer skin implies more blood flow and is a sign of a relaxed state. Temperature biofeedback deals with controlling autonomic arousal. In general, raising finger temperature indicates lowering of arousal, while decreasing the temperature indicates increases in arousal. In evaluating the progress of the use of this method, the amount and degree to which the patient can consistently control finger temperature should be emphasized, rather than comparing patient's performance to norms. Special instruments are used to monitor skin temperature and feed information back to the patient.

Electromyographic Feedback

There are two modes of electromyographic biofeedback (EMG BF): passive for reducing muscle activity (relaxation), and active for learning efficient use of muscles. In the passive mode, where the patient sits or lies down, the technique is used to teach patients to reduce muscle tension. In the active mode, EMG BF is used to aid therapy and facilitate performance. For example, patients can be taught efficient use of muscles for proper body mechanics during general activities. Proper body mechanics is expected to produce a lower EMG level for a given task. Patients can also be taught to control muscle activity while performing specific exercise-oriented activity. The latter type of EMG BF application in the active mode is referred to as muscle reeducation.

MUSCLE REEDUCATION

Muscle reeducation (MR) is an approach where patients learn to use neuromuscular loop pathways that may have been blocked or inhibited by injury or pain. Alternatively, patients may be able to *chart* new pathways from the brain to the muscles. In low back pain patients MR may take the form of an exercise treatment modality that combines the principles of electromyographic biofeedback with a progressive back extension strengthening routine (Asfour et al., 1990).

FUNCTIONAL ELECTRICAL STIMULATION

Muscular strengthening can be accomplished through two modes of exercise: active (regular isometric or dynamic exercise) and passive (electrical stimulation). Active exercise sometimes places great demands on patients. Due to muscle weakness, some patients experience difficulty in attempting to perform regular *active* exercise designed to strengthen weak muscles. Moreover, since many chronic low back pain patients suffer considerable loss of strength and muscle bulk due to disuse and inactivity, their voluntary effort is diminished and more time than usual is needed to regain strength. It is, therefore, desirable to provide the CLBP patient with a method of strengthening key muscles of the legs through effective and less physiologically demanding exercises. Functional electrical stimulation (FES) has proved to provide reconditioning and restoration of function of weak muscles in a variety of conditions. As an added-on modality during rehabilitation, FES can help to expedite strength recovery without interfering with other medical conditions that might not allow the individual to perform active exercises. It has been shown that FES is effective in removal of muscle inhibition resulting from conversion, such as in the case of hysterical or conversion paralysis (Khalil, Abdel-Moty, Asfour, Fishbain, Rosomoff, and Rosomoff, 1988).

Functional electric stimulation deals with the control of skeletal movement through electric excitation of the neuromuscular system. It provides control of muscle fiber contraction in the target muscle through the excitation generated in the neural system. Many studies report the usefulness of electrical stimulation in a variety of cases. Examples of the reported applications are to restore ankle dorsiflexion during gait training (Turk and Kralj, 1980); to correct foot drop (Mereletti et al., 1979); to elicit functional movement in paralyzed muscles (Nemeth, 1982); to rehabilitate knee injuries (Bohannon, 1983); to reduce spasticity (Alfieri, 1982); to treat scoliosis (Herbert, 1983); to retard disuse atrophy during immobilization (Gould et al., 1982; Standish and Valiant, 1981); to improve strength and working capacity of normal muscles (Currier and Mann, 1983; Laughman and Youdas, 1983); to increase isometric muscle strength and improve muscle contraction (McMiken et al., 1983; Selkowitz, 1985); to increase isokinetic strength (Romero et al., 1982); to increase muscle girth (Godfrey et al., 1979); to restore muscle function in conversion paralysis patients (Khalil, Abdel-Moty, Asfour, Fishbain, Rosomoff, Rosomoff, 1988); and to improve muscular output in patients with chronic low back pain (Abdel-Moty et al., 1986).

Functional Electrical Stimulation in Low Back Pain Patients

The usefulness of functional electrical stimulation (FES) in the rehabilitation of chronic low back pain (CLBP) patients with identifiable muscle weakness has been documented earlier (Abdel-Moty, Khalil, Rosomoff, and Rosomoff, 1987, 1988b). Patients with CLBP exhibit significant weakness of lower extremity muscles, usually on one side compared to the other. This characteristic is common among CLBP patients, particularly those with primary or residual quadriceps paresis. Prolonged muscle disuse creates weakness, and in many cases atrophy. It also creates imbalance in the human posture and biomechanical instability. Injury and pain can also create a condition of total or partial conversion paralysis, which responds to FES treatment (Khalil, Abdel-Moty, Asfour, Fishbain, Rosomoff, Rosomoff, 1988).

Suggested Methods of Application

The following are suggested methods of functional electrical stimulation (FES) application to the quadriceps (Fig. 9.2):

1. Place large flexible conductive rubber stimulation electrodes over the weaker quadriceps muscle.

2. Secure electrodes with Velcro straps.

3. Align electrodes in a bipolar configuration along the length of the thigh.

Principles and Methods of Interventions   151

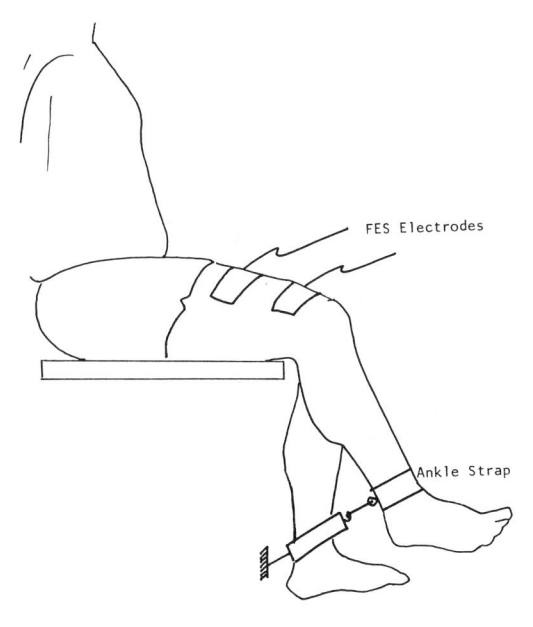

FIGURE 9.2.   Experimental task of knee extension and electrodes placement for FES application.

4. Place damp sponges between the electrodes and the skin to provide electric conductivity.

5. Apply the electric stimulus in a total of 15 bursts (15 seconds ON, followed by a 35-second OFF period before the next burst is applied). Increase the intensity of the stimulus gradually to the maximum tolerance of the individual.

6. Record the threshold of sensation and tolerance to stimulation.

7. Observe the quality of muscular contraction and response to stimulation.

8. Use quantitative measures of muscle strength, muscle mass (girth), electromyography, and ranges of motion to document neuromuscular response to treatment.

10

Principles and Methods of Interventions Through Work Conditioning and Work Hardening

It is important to raise the individual's tolerance levels so that he/she has adequate ability to perform tasks required in the work or home environment. This is accomplished through work conditioning and work hardening.

WORK CONDITIONING

The objective of *work conditioning* is to improve the patients' physical condition (flexibility, mobility, tolerance, strength, endurance) and to allow them to practice job tasks efficiently with proper posture and body mechanics. These goals should be accomplished under proper supervision. The ergonomist looks at the motions, time, and forces required to perform the tasks, so that physical task demands in relation to patients' abilities can be determined and matched. This is important to the total rehabilitation process, since identification of an individual's strengths and weaknesses can help the medical team orient the treatment program in the direction of full functional restoration. An essential part of work conditioning programs is job/task simulation. It should be understood that it is not possible, nor is it necessary, to replicate jobs. It is also not necessary to simulate a full working day of eight hours, unless a work tolerance evaluation is to be performed.

The structure of a work conditioning program may vary in intensity (two to eight hours per day), tasks performed (actual or simulated), and its components (standing, sitting, walking, climbing, lifting, etc.), personnel involved (medical, ergonomic), and in the approach to functional restoration (progressive nature of the work conditioning for individualized building up of tolerances and capacities).

Basically, work conditioning procedures consist of six main orderly steps designed to

- increase posture and body mechanics awareness,
- increase flexibility and mobility,
- increase strength and endurance,
- improve skill in managing stress, pain control, safety, and preventive medicine,
- modify behaviors toward work and employment,
- perform ergonomic job analysis and job simulation.

WORK HARDENING

Work hardening (WH) is a newly used name for traditional techniques of improving performance and endurance in industrial and rehabilitative service. In general, WH aims at improving function. In industry, WH is the equivalent of training or retraining workers in order to improve their abilities to carry out job tasks. For patients with low back pain, WH aims at maximizing the abilities of the injured worker in order to safely expedite a return to work. In 1988 the Commission on Accreditation of Rehabilitation Facilities (CARF) developed a set of standards and guidelines for the establishment and practice of WH programs. A primary difference between work conditioning and work hardening is that work hardening programs are, in general, not set up to handle patients requiring medical or psychological treatment. Usually, such individuals enter the WH programs following the appropriate clinical intervention. CARF defined WH as follows: "Work hardening is a highly structured, goal-oriented, individualized treatment program designed to maximize the individual's ability to return to work. Work hardening programs, which are interdisciplinary in nature, use real or simulated work activities in conjunction with conditioning tasks that are graded to progressively improve the biomechanical, neuromuscular, cardiovascular/metabolic, and psychosocial functions of the individual. Work hardening provides a transition between acute care and return to work, while addressing the issues of productivity, safety, physical tolerances, and worker behavior." Well-designed work hardening programs should be based on all the principles of ergonomics described earlier in this book.

11
Applications and Case Studies of Ergonomic Interventions

The following case presentations and examples demonstrate the use of the ergonomic interventions described in the previous chapters. In addition to the case studies, sample profiles are also presented in order to provide the statistical rationale for the generalization of results. The information presented is drawn from actual applications implemented by the authors at the University of Miami Comprehensive Pain and Rehabilitation Center (CPRC) and in other locations.

CASE STUDIES IN ERGONOMIC JOB ANALYSIS, POSTURE, AND BODY MECHANICS

Several cases were selected to represent some examples of the value of applying and implementing ergonomic job analysis and workplace/task design principles and guidelines for the reduction of stresses. In the cases presented, ergonomically inspired design solutions were applied to minimize the stresses due to poor engineering of the environment, task, tools, and the workplace in general.

CASE 1—Ergonomics in Dentistry

The work environment in a dental office represents a good example of a human-machine system (Fig. 11.1). The dentist interacts with equipment

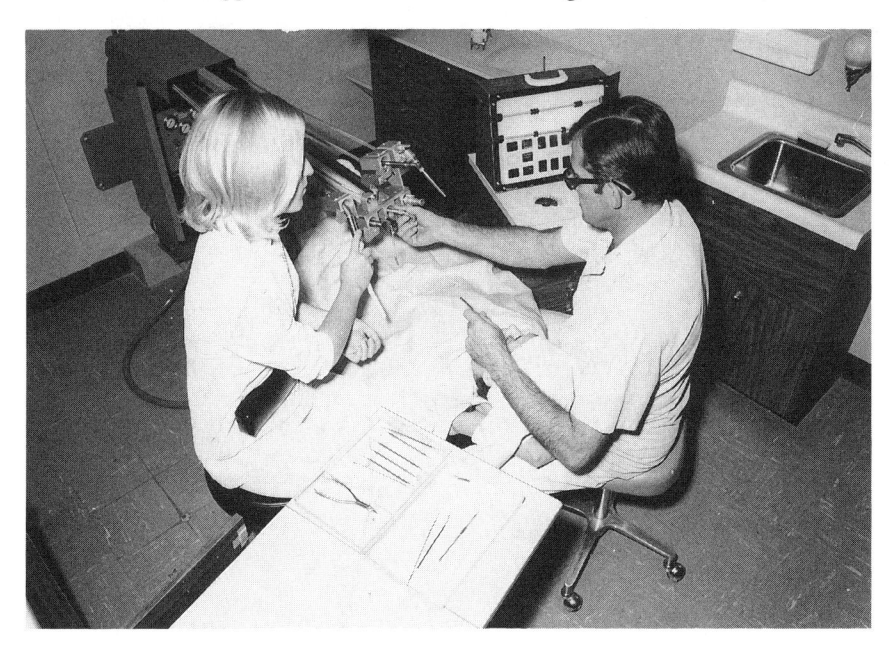

FIGURE 11.1. The dental practice workplace (Khalil and Truscheit, 1974).

and dental assistants to deliver services to a patient in the confines of the dental operatory environment. Dentists are known to suffer from low back pain, uneven shoulders, varicose veins, tension headaches, and eye strain. They also have one of the highest mortality rate of any professional group. Khalil (1974) and Khalil and Bell (1972, 1974) attribute many of these problems to the traditionally poor design of the dentist's equipment and work environment. Optimal arrangement of facilities and procedures can reduce static stresses, reduce fatigue, produce effective systems, and help increase work quality and quantity. Khalil and Bell (1972, 1974) suggest various ergonomic solutions to reduce stresses on the dentist's musculoskeletal system. Their implementation of an ergonomic approach to the redesign of the dental operatory system had significant impact on the design and operation of that system (Fig. 11.2). In this approach, the dental delivery system is described according to its configuration and dental unit locations. There is equipment in the rear, side, and front areas. The following are some of the criteria used to evaluate the system:

1. **Biomechanical Factors** availability of instruments, height of work surfaces, human posture, muscular force, and physiological expenditure

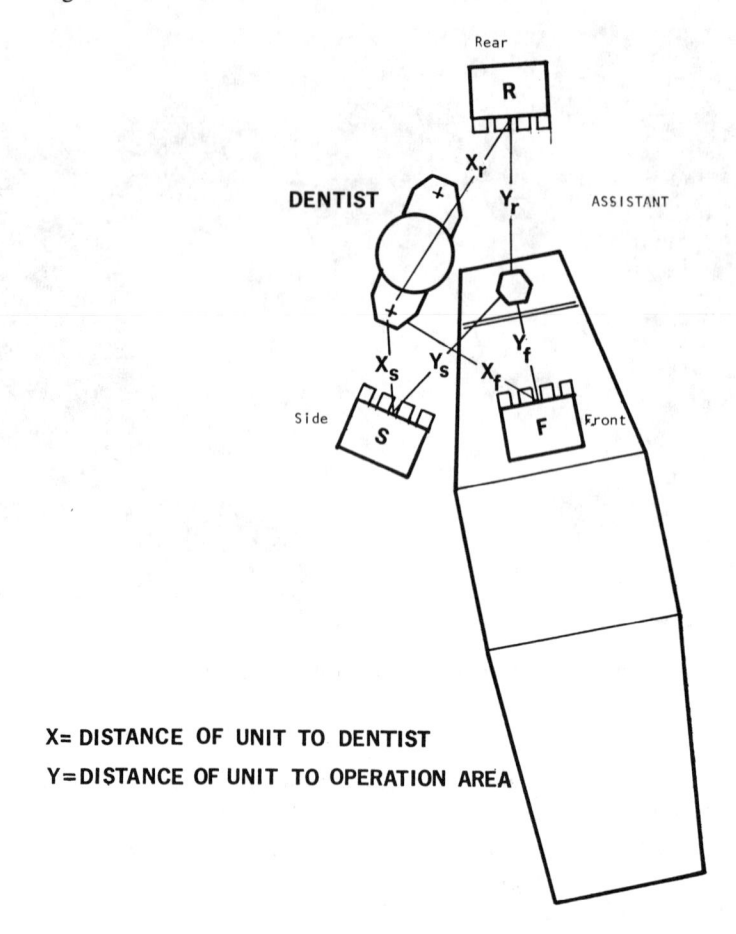

X= DISTANCE OF UNIT TO DENTIST
Y= DISTANCE OF UNIT TO OPERATION AREA

FIGURE 11.2. Ergonomic intervention in the dental delivery system consisted of studying and modifying the total environment in which the dentist and the assistant work in order to optimize reaches in all directions and minimize unnecessary movement.

2. **Human Movement** requiring minimum time and minimum fatigue, and covering short distances
3. **Delays** those inherent in the delivery system and the clinical procedure, those due to inadequate operatory management, and those caused by the human component
4. **Time** per patient, per procedure, per involvement, to prepare for the following patient, and for equipment servicing
5. **Flexibility** for sit/stand operations, left/right hand operations, working with/without assistant, and the need to perform all facets of dentistry

6. **Hygiene** in terms of ease of maintenance of equipment, walls, floors, parts, etc.
7. **Safety** of the patients and the therapy team

In order to ensure the proper design of the work system, ergonomic principals were implemented as follows:

1. For manual control areas the 1st percentile values were selected to accommodate the shortest subjects, and for space requirements the 95th percentile was selected to accommodate the largest person.

2. There should be standardization and effective training of all personnel.

3. Hand instruments should be properly designed to be compatible with human anatomy and physiology.

4. Restructure the task to permit compatibility.

5. Adjust illumination, noise, vibration, and temperature levels.

Khalil and Bell (1972, 1974) indicate that the principles of ergonomics can have a significant impact on the design and operation of the dental health care delivery system and advocate the implementation of ergonomic principles and concepts during the design stage. The use of sit down posture by the dentist and the proper ergonomically inspired design of the environment, reduce stress on the dentist. It contributes to the reduction of low back pain and other occupationally induced health problems.

CASE 2—Electrician

This is the case of a 43-year-old male. He works as a commercial electrician for an electric company. His work duties include bending pipes, hanging pipes, installing junction boxes, pulling wires, climbing ladders wearing a 30-pound tool belt on the right hip, and trouble shooting. He also reads and rewrites blueprints. He sustained an injury to the lower back, was rehabilitated, and returned to work. Ergonomic interventions consisted of modifying the design of the tool used for bending pipes in such a way that allows better use of stronger muscles, better mechanical advantage, and certainly reduced stresses on the low back (Fig. 11.3).

CASE 3—a Photojournalist

This is a 35-year-old male who sustained a cumulative trauma-type injury. Pain was in right lower extremity, mostly at the hip. No specific incident

158 Ergonomics in Back Pain

(A) Before Modification   (B) Modified Design

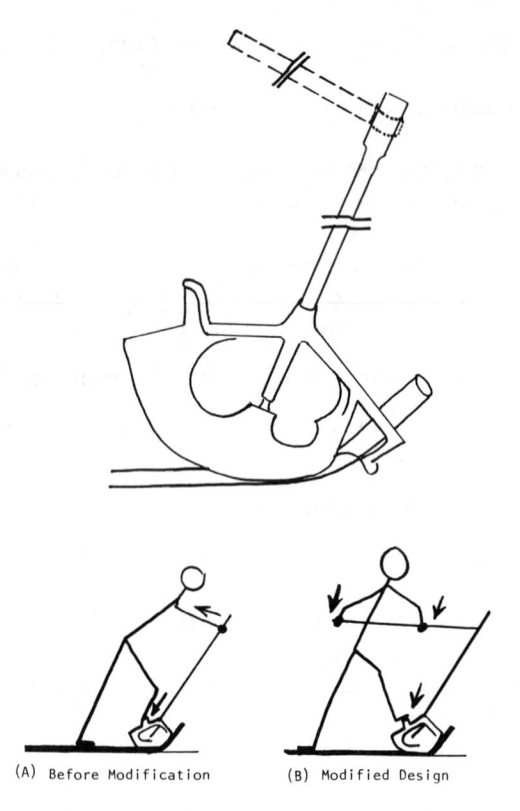

FIGURE 11.3. An ergonomic modification to the design of a pipe bending work tool. The new design reduces stress on the back and the chances of low back pain.

was identified as the cause of pain. He reported that pain developed gradually. He is a photojournalist. His job consists of photographing news, events, locations, illustrative and educational material; using still cameras; and carrying a tool bag, and suitcase. Biomechanical analysis showed the pain condition could be attributed to the uneven weight distribution due to carrying the tools for extended periods of time each day (Fig. 11.4A). The intervention in this case was the design of a vest that could be used to contain all work objects in a manner that allowed ease of access and even distribution of weight on the hips. The new design permits more force balance on the body parts, thus restoring biomechanical balance (Fig. 11.4B). The introduction of the new design was estimated to reduce the biomechanical forces on the L5/S1 joint by about 30%, while back muscle forces were reduced by 42%. Proper posture was maintained and discomfort was significantly reduced.

Applications and Case Studies of Ergonomic Interventions   159

(a) External Loads Before Modification.

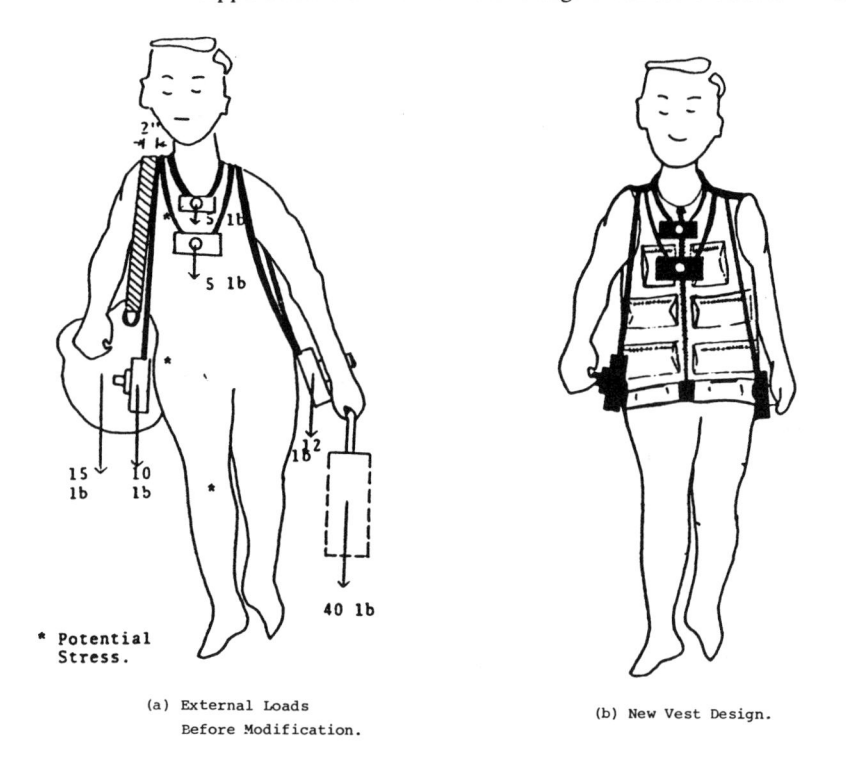

(b) New Vest Design.

FIGURE 11.4. Biomechanical analysis showed high stress levels at the neck, hip, knee, and the lower back of a photojournalist due to static, uneven loading. Ergonomic intervention involved the design of a special vest and redistribution of external load (Abdel-Moty, Khalil, Asfour et al., 1988).   *Stress location identified via biomechanical analysis and reported by the patient.

CASE 4—Musical Conductor

This is a 69-year-old musical conductor. He had several years of intermittent low back and leg pain. Job requirements include selecting, scheduling, directing, and conducting symphony orchestras for up to three hours. While being treated at the pain center, job simulation was performed. He brought musical notes and a stand. He simulated a live performance while being videotaped. His posture, low back muscle activity, ranges of motion, and heart rate were monitored continuously during a 90-minute simulation. Risk factors were identified as angle of vision, body weight shift, feet separation, twisting, and bending. This resulted in an 88% increase in heart rate and a 33 uV*sec level of EMG. Intervention consisted of reviewing and analyzing the videotape in order to identify problems and suggest

160   Ergonomics in Back Pain

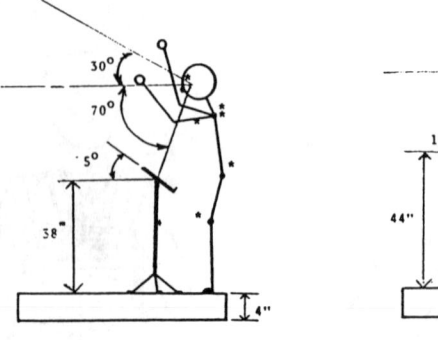

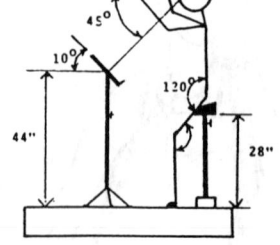

(a) Before Modification   (b) After Modifications

FIGURE 11.5. Changes in body posture and enviornmental design after ergonomic intervention with this orchestra conductor (Abdel-Moty, Khalil, Asfour et al., 1988).

solutions. Recommendations for proper body mechanics were offered in order to reduce muscle tension (pelvic tilt, leveling of shoulders, aligning of head and neck, widening of base of support, proper turning of the body, etc.). In order to reduce muscle tension and static loading further during prolonged standing, a high stool was designed (Fig. 11.5). This allowed semi-standing/sitting posture whenever fatigue was experienced. This chair was adjustable, had a slight angle at the seat, and had soft cushioning. The combined ergonomic intervention decreased EMG of the paraspinals by 140% and allowed only a 46% increase in heart rate following a 90-minute simulation session.

CASE 5—Radiologist

This is a 41-year-old male radiologist. He complained of shoulders, neck, buttocks, and thigh pains. He reported increased pain, muscle cramping, and numbness following physical activity, especially weight-bearing. His job required wearing a 15-pound lead apron for about eight hours daily. At the pain center, ergonomists analyzed back and neck force biomechanically and recommended appropriate measures. Analysis showed that the lead apron placed 300 lb. inch of torque on the low back region, not to mention the static loading of the neck, arms, shoulders, and upper back. Recommendations included the redesign of the apron in order to allow distribution of weight, less static stresses, and less static loading (Fig. 11.6). Biomechanical forces on the low back were reduced by more than 80%, and posture was improved significantly.

Applications and Case Studies of Ergonomic Interventions 161

(A) Before Modification   (B) After Modification

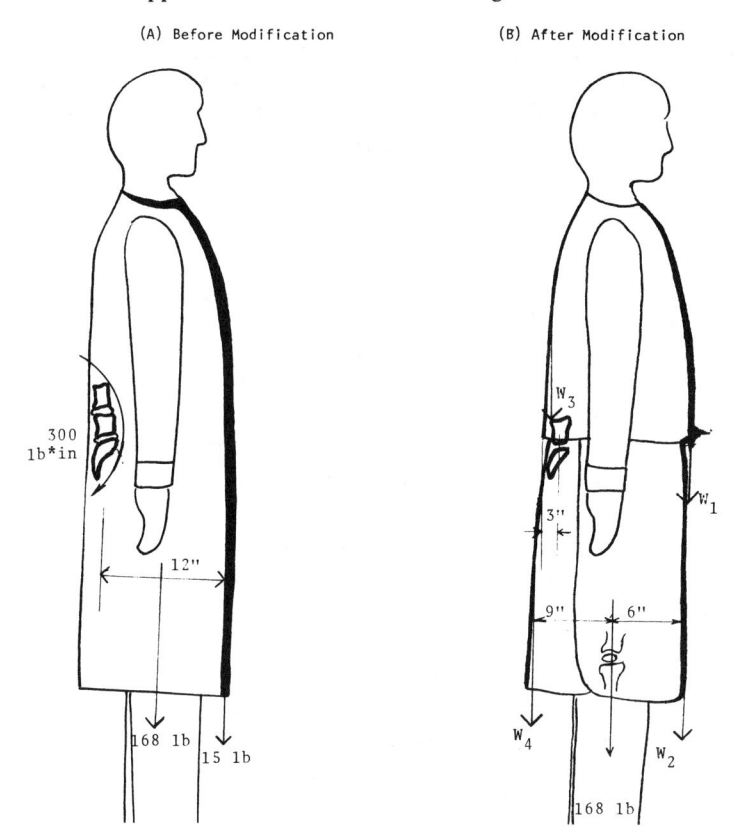

FIGURE 11.6. Apron design and moments on the low back before and after ergonomic intervention for a radiologist. New design of the apron balanced the weight distribution (Abdel-Moty, Khalil, Asfour et al., 1988).

CASE 6—The Sitting Workplace (from Abdel-Moty, Khalil, Goldberg et al., 1990)

This is a 42-year-old female. She is a research scientist (biochemist) with a state university. She is right-handed, stands 65 inches tall, weighs 128 pounds, and uses eyeglasses. In 1973 she began to develop episodes of LBP, with pain extending down the left leg (no accident involved). She was treated with bedrest for two weeks. In 1979 she developed right LBP, which remained intermittent thereafter for several months. Pain was increased by activity. In 1983 she had a major exacerbation, with pain bilaterally in the low back, again treated with bedrest and medications. In 1987 she received physiotherapy two times a week for six weeks. In 1988 she entered the CPRC for evaluation and treatment. Upon admission, she reported pain in the low back and left leg. She reflected:

"Pain is almost constant in low back—both sides hurt but not together. When pain is on the right side then right knee and arch of right foot hurt; when pain is on left side, calf and heel of left leg hurt. Activity involving standing increases the pain. Back pain usually is not *bad* at night. I start the day relatively fine but it (the pain) gets worse as the day goes on. I would like to be able to stand up and play tennis again!"

She clearly recognized that she has been depressed and angry.

Initial neurological examination showed normal gait, good equilibrium and coordination, intact motor and sensory system, equal and active reflexes bilaterally, good ranges of back motion, tenderness over the right ischial tuberosity, and tight hamstring and hip rotators. The impression gathered was that there was no evidence of active nerve root compression, no surgical indications. She was given the diagnosis of lumbar myofascial syndrome, the type of condition that responds to an aggressive physical medicine program to which she has not been exposed to prior to her admission to the CPRC. Upon admission to the rehabilitation program at the CPRC, her treatment program consisted of physical therapy, occupational therapy, vocational rehabilitation, behavioral modification, detoxification, and ergonomic consultation for functional capacity assessment (FCA) and ergonomic job analysis (EJA) (Rosomoff et al., 1981; Khalil et al., 1983).

Ergonomics job analysis methods described in Chapter 4 were utilized. In the *data collection* phase and during the first week of the patient's admission to the treatment, an initial evaluation was performed in order to obtain both individual and job-related information. The following were components of this evaluation:

1. Basic biographic information and physical characteristics of the individual: age, weight, height, occupation, cause and course of injury, and employment status. A summary of this information was given previously.

2. Qualitative description of the physical environment within which the job was performed: In this category the layout of the workplace and equipment parameters (locations, dimensions, priorities, frequency of use, etc.) were obtained through patient's description. She was asked to obtain photographs of the work environment;

3. Patient's self-description of a *typical* work day: From this description, job tasks were identified, the average time required to perform each task was estimated, and the sequence of tasks performance was determined. She described the day as follows: meeting with staff, writing and typing, telephone calls in one office, word processing and data analysis in another office, in addition to general laboratory activities.

Tasks were classified as follows:

Overall:
sitting   60%   standing   30%
walking   10%

While Sitting:
writing   30%   typing   10%   meeting   5%
talking on the phone   10%   working with VDT   40%
Viewing cells using microscope   5%

While Standing and Walking:
reaching   30%   lifting   10%   carrying   20%
Other lab activities   40%

An *initial evaluation* was then performed with the purpose of analyzing patient's performance, especially muscular work. At this stage, the job (the physical environment as well as the task) was simulated and assessment was performed as follows:

1. Task/job simulation: The information gathered from the initial evaluation was used, in conjunction with the patient's input, to construct a workplace that closely simulates the actual work station. It was recognized that exact reproduction of the environment is impossible since there are many factors (heat, noise, fumes, etc.) that are difficult to emulate. The goal here was to analyze the patient's patterns of movement (body mechanics) within the environment. The bench, the office, and the computer workstations were simulated.

2. Analysis of Task Performance: In order to evaluate the manner in which the patient performed job tasks prior to admission to the CPRC, the patient performed tasks in the simulated environment that were similar to those encountered on the job. Emphasis was on activities that were done repeatedly or for long periods of time, such as VDT tasks, viewing the microscope, talking on the phone, doing regular desk tasks, and performing bench-type activities (sampling, test tubes, mixing compounds, etc.). The goal was to identify the tasks that contributed more to stress production. For objective evaluation of performance, electrical activity of the lower back muscles were recorded (see section A of Fig. 11.7). No feedback or suggestions for modifications or adjustments were given at this stage. Patient's self-report of discomfort/pain at the beginning and end of this 30-minute evaluation session were obtained. Overall, she reported an in-

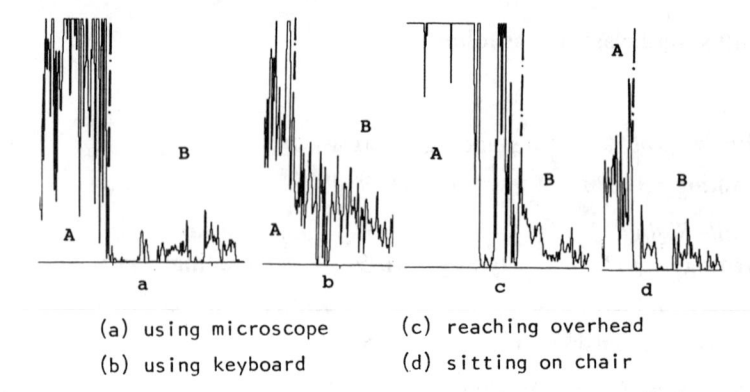

(a) using microscope (c) reaching overhead
(b) using keyboard   (d) sitting on chair

FIGURE 11.7. Electromyographic recording of right lumbar paraspinal muscles of a patient performing job tasks (a to d) prior to (A) and following (B) ergonomic job anlysis and intervention (Abdel-Moty, Khalil, Goldberg et al., 1990).

crease in pain level from an initial 6/10 to about 9/10 at the end of this session. The overall average EMG level during this simulation was 4.2 uV*sec.

3. Identification of the Risk Factors: While the simulated tasks were being performed, the evaluator observed patient's body mechanics and postural adjustment, identified critical motion patterns, and detected any mismatch between the patient's physical characteristics and the dimensions of the workplace. Also, levels of EMG activity were correlated with the different movements. The following were identified as potential problem areas: Inadequate elbow rest and chair parameters in general while sitting, work surface and keyboard heights relative to elbow height, lack of footrest while sitting or standing, neck postures while using the microscope and while on the phone, overreaching to cabinet, posture while sitting on a high stool to work at the bench, and VDT screen height.

Following the identification of the risk factors, the intervention included the following strategies:

1. Reengineering the Workplace: Sitting heights were adjusted based on anthropometric dimensions of the individual and work surface height; the layout of the workstation was modified so that all tools were within functional reaches; additional equipment (footrest, keyboard holder, three-step ladder to assist in reaching) were recommended in order to compensate for major deficiencies. The parameters of the VDT and other tools were adjusted according to the patient's capabilities. The expert system SWAD was used to supplement the design and analysis process so that proper seating parameters are determined for *her* anthropometric dimensions (Abdel-Moty and Khalil, 1986, a, b, 1987, a, b). Patient was given detailed information about the rationale of the modifications made.

2. Postural Adjustment: Provided that the physical match between the individual and the workplace was attained, the next step was to increase postural awareness. Principles of proper posture were implemented (Abdel-Moty et al., 1988c). It was important at this point to demonstrate to the patient, through EMG feedback, that these postural correction techniques do indeed reduce muscular tension and static stresses.

3. Body Mechanics Modification: Body movement at the workstation was corrected in order to minimize awkward patterns and reduce stresses resulting from activities such as twisting, overreaching and repetitive bending.

4. Learning and Practicing: The patient was then given the opportunity to practice the new techniques and appreciate their efficacy in providing stress reduction. Simulations were repeated and body mechanics were refined. Most often this type of activity was performed as a joint effort between ergonomics, occupational therapy, vocational rehabilitation, and biofeedback. The patient was taught to review work activities, execute her job tasks properly, receive suggestions for modifications or adjustments, and implement recommendations in the simulated environment. All these activities assured the patient that she would be capable of carrying them out when she returned to the actual work site.

The impact of these adjustments, modifications, and education on the muscle activity of the lumbar paraspinals muscles is shown in Figure 11.8 and is summarized in Table 11.1. No doubt, there was dramatic reduction in muscle work with the application of each intervention strategy.

A second evaluation was performed in order to determine, quantitatively, the changes in the outcome measures (EMG and self-report of pain) as a result of intervention. This evaluation session lasted 30 minutes and is reflected on the B section of Figure 11.7. The overall average EMG value was 0.95 uV*sec reflecting a tremendous reduction in muscle activity as compared to the initial average level (4.2 uV*sec) while performing the same tasks (Fig. 11.8). The combination of intervention and learning new techniques has allowed the patient to work at much lower physiological demand in the same environment. Furthermore, she reported no significant change in pain level at the end of the final evaluation session (initial evaluation increased pain by 50%).

166 Ergonomics in Back Pain

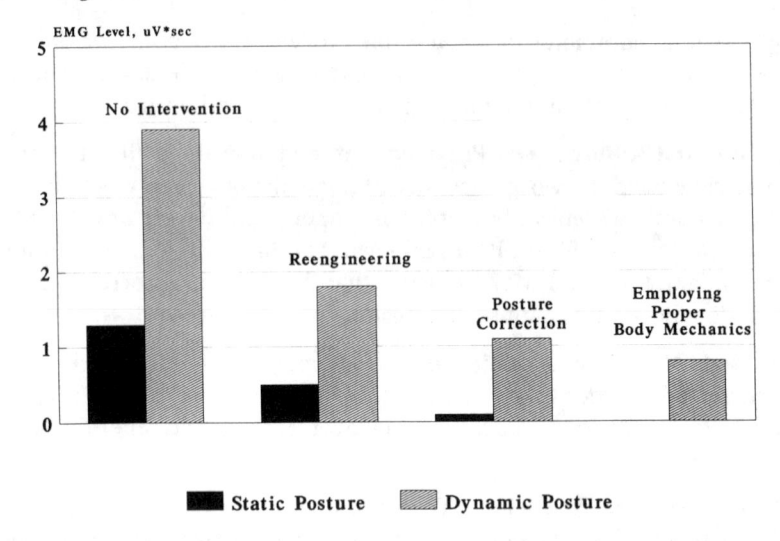

FIGURE 11.8. Average EMG levels recorded from the paraspinal muscles during static and dynamic postures upon administration of the various stages of EJA. Reengineering of the environment reduced muscle tension significantly. Further reduction was achieved through postural correction and proper body mechanics during activity (Abdel-Moty, Khalil, Goldberg et al., 1990).

TABLE 11.1 Average Level of the Electromyographic Activity of the Right Lumbar Paraspinal Muscles During Two types of Activities* (From Abdel-Moty, Khalil, Goldberg et al., 1990)

	Average Static[†]	EMG Level Dynamic[‡]
No Intervention	1.3	3.9
Reengineering of the workplace	0.5	1.6
Correcting posture	0.1	1.1
Employing proper body mechanics	NA[§]	0.9

*In micro volt/sec
[†]Static: Assuming selected work posture, no tasks performed.
[‡]Dynamic: Performing job tasks.
[§]NA: Condition not applicable.

BIOMECHANICS

Biomechanical models can be used for the analysis of job tasks. In an analysis of lifting tasks performed by nurses (Khalil, Asfour, Marchette, and Omachonu, 1987, and Khalil and Ramadan, 1987), biomechanical analysis using a static model was conducted. The method entailed photographing the nurses in various postures during a lifting task, analyzing the photographs, and calculating the biomechanical stresses exerted on the lumbar area. Analysis also required information such as the weight of the patient (load), weight of the nurse(s), anthropometric dimension of the nurse(s), and the distance between patient and the nurse. Analysis revealed the impact of the various work postures on back stress. Three postures were analyzed.

1. **Posture 1**: two nurses lifting a patient from the supine position (Fig. 11.9)
2. **Posture 2**: two nurses lifting a seated patient from the edge of a bed
3. **Posture 3**: two nurses lifting a seated patient from a chair

Erector spinae muscle force and the forces on L5/S1 are summarized in the Table 11.2 and in Figures 11.10 and 11.11. It can be seen that these two nurses are indeed exposed to high levels of stress while performing these daily tasks. This study identified various factors that can contribute to low back pain in nurses, among which are the lack of knowledge of nurse's realistic physical capabilities, the failure to determine the true weight of the load to be lifted, the failure to summon the assistance of a co-worker, the failure to utilize mechanical lifting devices, and the use of improper lifting techniques. The study recommended the use of lifting aids, providing sufficient space for proper use of body mechanics, screening of personnel, and education. Computerized biomechanical models (Khalil and Ramadan, 1987) can be helpful in quickly analyzing the magnitude of stresses on the musculoskeletal structures as a result of specific posture or load. However,

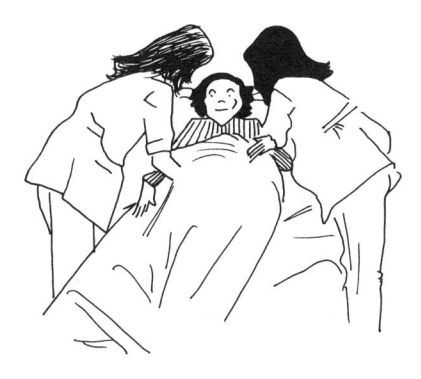

FIGURE 11.9. Nurses helping a patient to sit up in bed from a supine position. Stresses on the lower back were predicted by the biomechanical analysis being very high when the task is not properly performed (Khalil et al, 1987).

168   Ergonomics in Back Pain

TABLE 11.2   Biomechanical Stresses on Two Nurses for Various Postures (From Khalil, Asfour, Marchette, Omachonu, 1987).

	Nurse #1					Nurse #2				
Posture	Load Lifted	M	X	Y	R	Load Lifted	M	X	Y	R
#1	37.5	758	819	42	820	37.5	787	849	51	851
#2	50.0	515	616	72	620	50.0	536	634	71	638
#3	60.0	618	736	66	739	60.0	637	741	59	743

Notes:
Weight of Nurse #1 = 112 lb.
Weight of Nurse #2 = 107 lb.
M = Muscle tension force.
X = horizontal component of the force.
Y = Vertical component of the force.
R = Resultant force of X and Y.

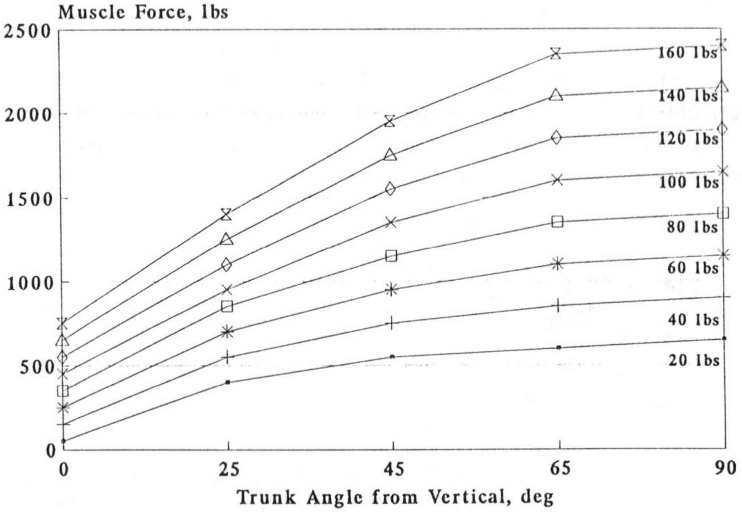

FIGURE 11.10.   Muscular force (lbs) versus trunk angle (deg) for different loads (from khalil et al., 1987).

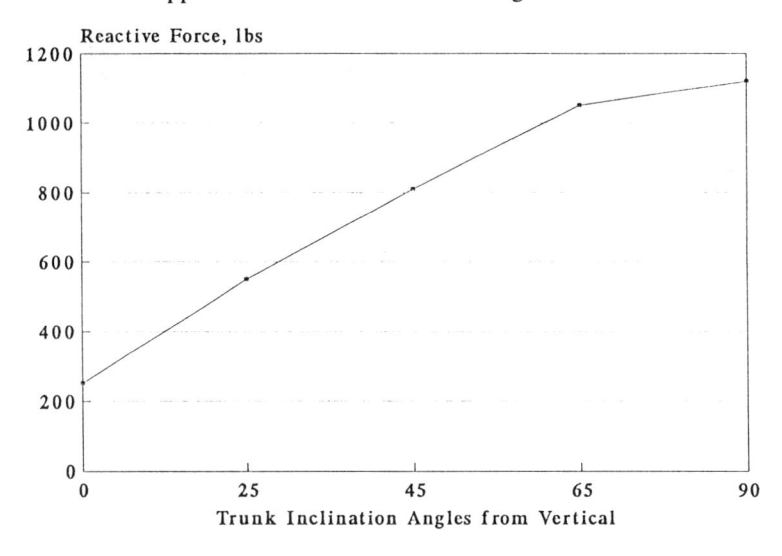

FIGURE 11.11 Reactive force on L5/S1 (lbs) versus trunk Inclination Angle (deg) (from Khalil et al., 1987)

one should exercise caution in interpreting results of computerized models, since they have embedded assumptions that may not necessarily reflect real world situations.

EVALUATION OF HUMAN CHARACTERISTICS

CASE 1—Individual Profile

This is a case of a 22-year old female who works as an electrician. While carrying a box of tools she tripped over a cable and fell on the coccyx. She felt immediate lower and upper back pain. Upon admission to the CPRC, she underwent an initial ergonomic evaluation of functional abilities (Table 11.3). The performance profile showed a significant loss in her functional abilities: trunk ranges of motion were limited; strength values were lower than those for healthy individuals of the same age group; walking pace was slower than normal; and tolerances for sitting, standing, and ambulation were limited. After four weeks of aggressive therapy, she reported significant reduction in pain level. Final evaluation showed significant increases in all measures of functional ability. The most dramatic increase was in the upper extremity and back static strengths.

Quantitative evaluation of performance was quite helpful in revealing

TABLE 11.3 Human Performance Profile Showing the Changes in Measures of Functional Abilities for the Case Study (From Khalil, Abdel-Moty, Asfour et al., 1990).

Measure	Initial	Final	Change
1. Grip strength (lb.)	60	70	+17%
2. AME (lb)			
Composite	90	120	+33%
Leg	160	216	+35%
Shoulder	35	68	+94%
Arm	26	55	>+100%*
Back	42	127	>+100%*
3. Trunk flexion (deg.)	70	120	+71%
4. Walking speed (ft/sec)	5.9	6.5	+11%
5. Functional tolerances			
Sitting (min.)	25	60	>+100%*
Standing (min.)	25	60	>+100%*
Ambulation (ft/min)	167	176	+5.4%
6. Reaction time (sec.)			
Simple	0.29	0.23	+26%
Choice	0.70	0.52	+35%
7. Hand steadiness (no.)	10	4	+60%
8. Squatting Ability (in.)	15	0	>+100%*
9. Posture score	85	95	+12%
10. Reported pain level	7	1	

* 100% is assigned to improvements of higher than double the initial value.

areas of weakness and establish a baseline from which progress after rehabilitation could be measured.

Another case study is presented in Figure 11.12 for a 40-year-old male who underwent a one-time functional capacity assessment in order to determine his vocational potential. As can be seen, findings were very useful in determining physical capabilities in reference to the Dictionary of Occupational Titles's 20 job factors. Information obtained through this type of evaluation can be used to suggest further physical/vocational preparation.

CASE 2—Population Profile

In order to determine the overall effectiveness of rehabilitation programs, population progress profiles can be established and then compared. The profile of a sample of 265 low back pain patients, classified as worker's compensation who were treated and completed the program at the CPRC, was established (Table 11.4). All patients underwent full ergonomic evaluations to determine their functional abilities and progress throughout the

Applications and Case Studies of Ergonomic Interventions 171

UNIVERSITY OF MIAMI
COMPREHENSIVE PAIN AND REHABILITATION CENTER

ERGONOMIC FUNCTIONAL CAPACITY ASSESSMENT
SUPPLEMENTAL EVALUATIONS

Name: G.D.M. Date: 2/22/1992

Age: 40 Sex: Male Weight: 210 lbs Height: 70" Dominant Hand: Right

Measurement	Score	Measurement	Score
Pain Level (0-10) Location	7 Head	Hand Steadiness (#)	10
Reaction Time (sec) Simple Visual Simple Auditory Choice	0.31 0.20 0.46	Squatting Ability (in)	0
		Walking Pace (ft/sec)	2.5
Anterior-Posterior Sway Eyes Opened Eyes Closed	Unable (Dizzy)	Lateral Sway Eyes Opened Eyes Closed	Unable (Dizzy)
Ranges of Motion (deg) a. Trunk Flexion Extension Lateral Right Lateral Left b. Cervical Flexion Extension Lateral Right Lateral Left	86/86/85 33/30/31 46/55/56 39/36/39 56/66/69 63/56/69 46/43/41 34/34/35	Static Strength (lb) Grip Right Left Arm AME Shoulder AME Composite AME Back AME Knee Ext. Right Left	92/90/87 70/72/69 144/151/106 198/166/126 192/154/175 Unable (Dizzy) 77/76/80 55/65/60

ERGONOMIC FUNCTIONAL CAPACITY ASSESSMENT - DOT FACTORS

DOT Job Factor	Score or Check Right	Left	WN	Reason for Stopping/Unable
Sitting tolerance	60 min		Y	
Feeling shapes	Able		Y	
Feeling sizes	Able		Y	
Feeling temperature	Able		Y	
Feeling texture	Able		Y	
Picking	Able		Y	
Tip pinching	13.5 lb.	12.2 lb.	Y	
Key pinching	14.6 lb.	11.7 lb.	Y	
Palmar pinching	15.0 lb.	12.2 lb.	Y	
Handling seizing	Able	Able	Y	
Handling holding	Able	Able	Y	
Handling grasping	Able	Able	Y	
Handling turning	Unable	Able	N/Y	Right wrist surgery/pain
Reaching standing	180 deg.	180 deg.	Y	

FIGURE 11.12. Ergonomic functional capacity assessment profile of a 40 year old male describing performance in various physical, functional, and DOT job factors.

172 Ergonomics in Back Pain

DOT Job Factor	Score or Check	WDN	Reason for Stopping/Unable
Stooping	86 deg.	Y	
Kneeling	Able	Y	
Crouching	Able	Y	
Crawling	Able	Y	
Balancing standing	Unable	N	Reported feeling dizzy
Balancing walking	Able	Y	
Balancing crouching	Able	Y	
Standing tolerance	30 min.	Y	
Walking tolerance	2.5 miles, 120 min.	Y	
Climbing	Able	Y	
Pushing	175 lb.	Y	
Pulling	175 lb.	Y	
Carrying	0 lb.	N	Refused following lifting
Lifting	80 lb.	Y	

COMMENTS: Right wrist fusion, "fatigues by time."
Right index finger surgery.
Reported feeling dizzy several times during testing.

WDN : Within Defined Norms (Yes/No)

FIGURE 11.12. *(Continued)*

four-week rehabilitation program. Sample characteristics are also presented.

Results of the initial and final evaluations reflected statistically significant changes in the physical capacities of the patients (Table 11.5) and restoration of strength abilities to levels recorded for a healthy population, sometimes referred to as "norms" (Fig. 11.13). The improvement in static

TABLE 11.4   Descriptive Data for a Sample of 265 Low Back Pain Patients

Number of males	179
Number of females	86
Average age	42
Occupation:	
Heavy	36%
Moderate work	30%
Light work	34%
Cause of injury:	
Falls	42%
Lifting and carrying	25%
Auto accidents	8%
Simple bending	5%
Struck-by	5%
Pushing and pulling	8%
Other	8%

Applications and Case Studies of Ergonomic Interventions 173

TABLE 11.5 Human Performance Profile: Summary of Statistics (sample-size = 265)

Measure	Initial	Final
Trunk Flexion (deg.)	79.1	117.5
Composite AME (lb)	75.7	172.1
Leg AME (lb)	98.2	209.1
Shoulder AME (lb)	41.7	73.0
Arm AME (lb)	41.5	69.5
Walking pace (ft/sec)	3.4	5.0

strength was associated with pain reduction for both males and females (Figs. 11.14, 11.15). Additionally, other measures of functional abilities did change, reflecting improvement (Figs. 11.16 through 11.19). This is clearly manifested in the measures of the trunk ranges of motion and static strength. Quantitative measurements made by ergonomists have provided a quantitative way of evaluating the outcome of the rehabilitation treatment that these patients have undergone.

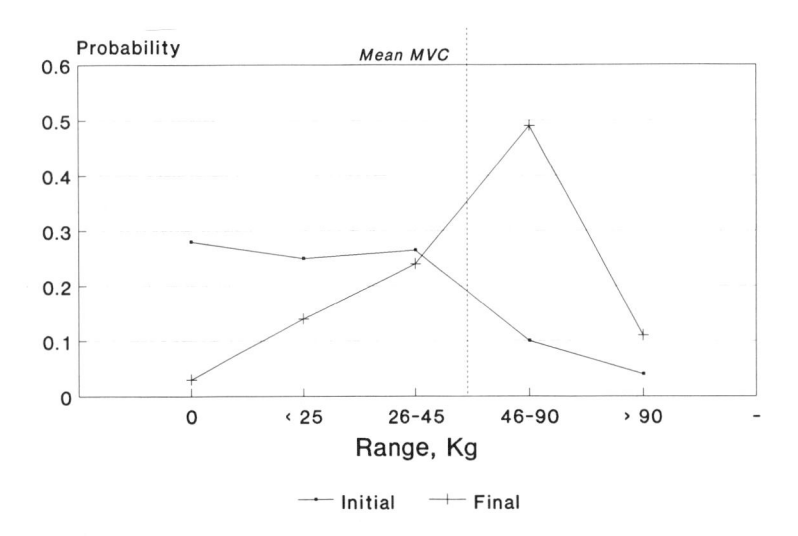

FIGURE 11.13. Prior to treatment (initial evaluation), the probability distribution of AME was skewed to the left, indicating a higher percentage of patients displaying low strength scores. Post-rehabilitation (final evaluation), the probability distribution was shifted to the right, indicating that AME values approached and exceeded norms for healthy subjects.

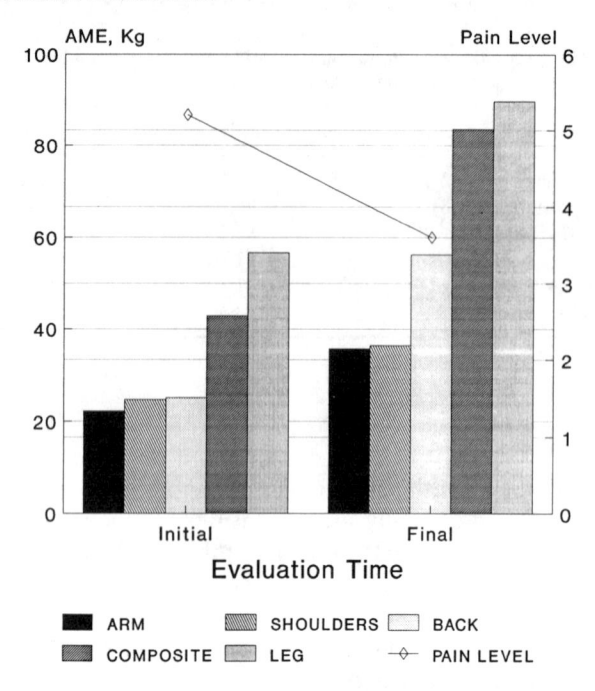

FIGURE 11.14. Initial and final AME for the various testing postures prior to and following rehabilitation of 100 male chronic low back pain patients. Findings reflect significant physical improvement associated with self-report of pain reduction.

ELECTROMYOGRAPHY

CASE 1—EMG for Quantifying Effectiveness of FES

A patient sustained an injury to the lower back when he slipped and twisted his body. As part of his physical conditioning program, he received functional electrical stimulation (FES) to restore function to the right ankle dorsiflexion muscles. Measures of muscle performance (strength, girth, range of joint motion) were used in conjunction with surface recorded EMG of the tibialis anterior to quantify treatment outcome. Evaluations were performed prior to treatment and after two weeks. Results are presented in Table 11.6.

It can clearly be seen that there was a drastic loss in muscle function before treatment. The strength of the right dorsiflexors was only five pounds, as compared to the strong performance of the left side (MVC = 30 lb). Meanwhile, EMG activity of the right tibialis anterior muscle was very depressed. EMG amplitude measures showed approximately a 1:10 ratio between the recruitment level of the right and left tibialis anterior muscles.

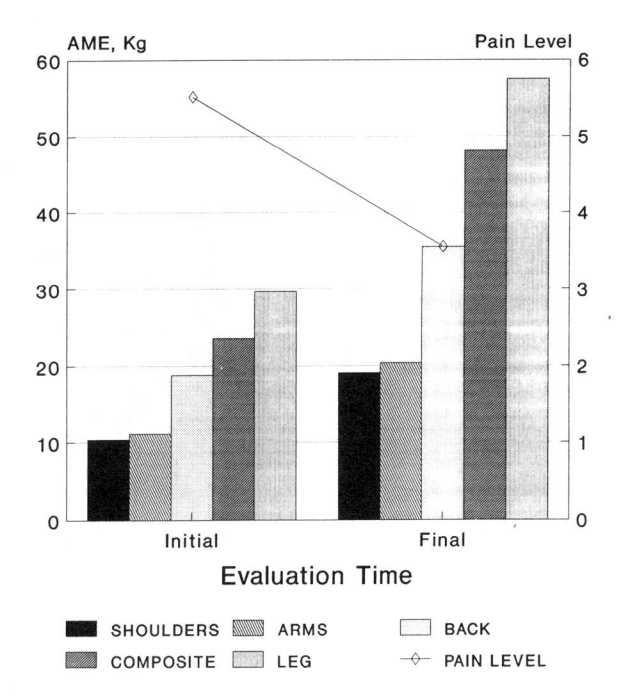

FIGURE 11.15. Initial and final AME for the various testing postures prior to and following rehabilitation of 98 female chronic low back pain patients. Findings reflect significant physical improvement associated with self-report of pain reduction.

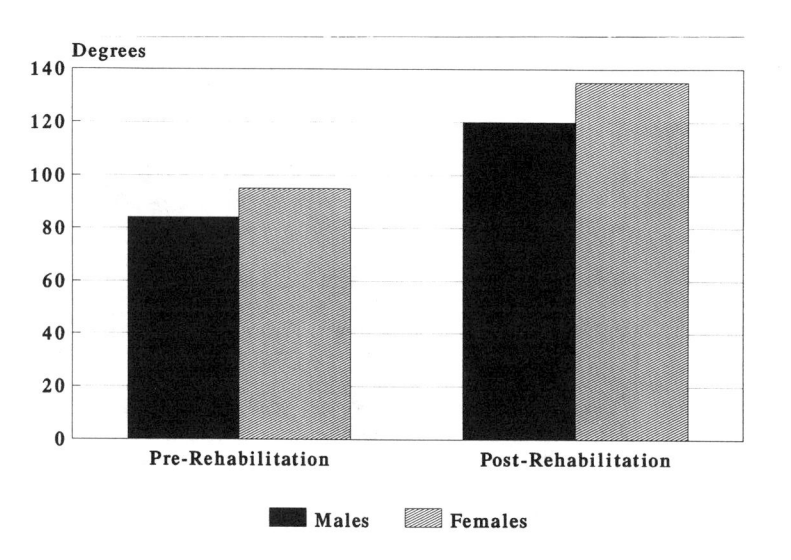

* Statistically Significant at 0.05

FIGURE 11.16. Improvement in trunk flexion ranges of motion of 200 patients with chronic low back pain.

* Statistically Significant at 0.05

FIGURE 11.17. Improvement in trunk extension range of motion of 230 patients with chronic low back pain.

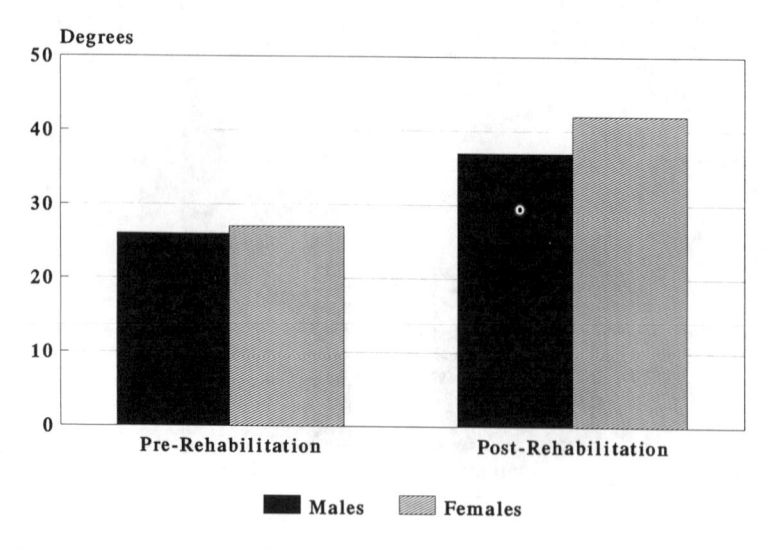

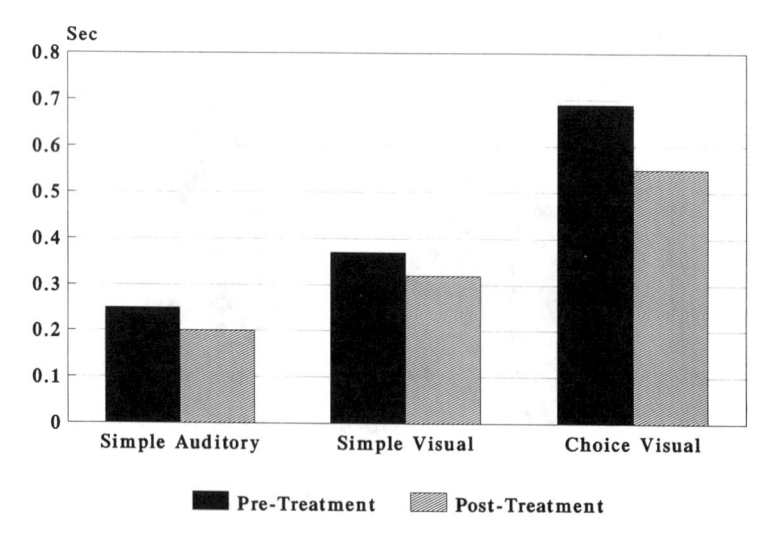

* Statistically Significant at 0.05

FIGURE 11.18. Effect of rehabilitation on functional restoration can also be found in patients' increased ability to respond to a stimuli.

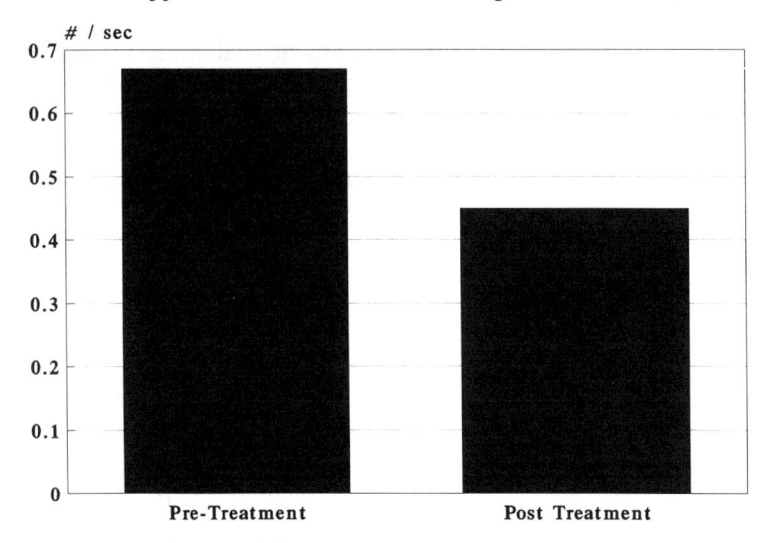

Applications and Case Studies of Ergonomic Interventions 177

```
     # / sec
0.7 ┌────────────────────────────────────┐
    │ ███████████                        │
0.6 │ ███████████                        │
    │ ███████████                        │
0.5 │ ███████████                        │
    │ ███████████    ███████████         │
0.4 │ ███████████    ███████████         │
    │ ███████████    ███████████         │
0.3 │ ███████████    ███████████         │
    │ ███████████    ███████████         │
0.2 │ ███████████    ███████████         │
    │ ███████████    ███████████         │
0.1 │ ███████████    ███████████         │
  0 └─────────────────────────────────────┘
      Pre-Treatment   Post Treatment
```

* Statistically Significant at 0.05

FIGURE 11.19. Improvement in hand steadiness upon rehabilitation of a sample of 50 chronic low back pain.

The power spectrum of the surface EMG also showed a significant reduction of the energy contents in the EMG signal at all frequency bands. At the end of the two weeks of administering FES, strength and EMG values showed dramatic increases. Isometric muscle strength of the weak right dorsiflexors approached that of the stronger healthy left side. The EMG of

TABLE 11.6 Summary of Measures of Strength and Muscle Activities for the Tibilais Anterior Muscles of Case #3 (From Abdel-Moty, Khalil et al., 1987).

	Right		Left	
Measure	Initial	Final	Initial	Final
1. Maximum voluntary contraction (lb)	5	32	30	36
2. Calf girth (cm)	35	37.2	38	38
3. Mean rectified (mV)	5.9	33.1	51.7	53.5
4. Full wave rectified integral (mV/sec)	23.0	128.4	200.3	214.7
5. Energy (mV*mV)	26.9	735.2	821.7	856.0
6. Sum of voltage excursions (mV)	23.7	132.5	206.6	261.3
7. Number of amplitudes	122	466	1592	1426
8. Number of turning points	1155	1414	1592	1426
9. Band Width (Hz)	102.8	118.3	134.35	128.0
10. Median frequency (Hz)	62.5	58.6	31.5	35.2
11. Average firing frequency (Hz)	91.4	113.3	113.8	113.1

178   Ergonomics in Back Pain

the right tibialis anterior resembled that of a normal interference pattern. Measures of the amplitude contents of the EMG signal during the final evaluation showed more than a 400% increase in value when compared to those obtained during the initial evaluation. Also, there were changes in the measures of the frequency component of the myoelectric signals indicating increased firing of the motor units. The patient went on to finish his pain rehabilitation program successfully.

CASE 2—EMG for Assessing Workplace Design

Khalil (1973) developed a method for multiple recording and analysis of EMG signals from different sites (Fig. 11.20). This method of total integrated muscular activity (TIMA) allows quantitative evaluation of the EMG and muscle response to work tasks. Recording of individual muscle activities can also be useful in task analysis. Figures 11.21a and 11.21b

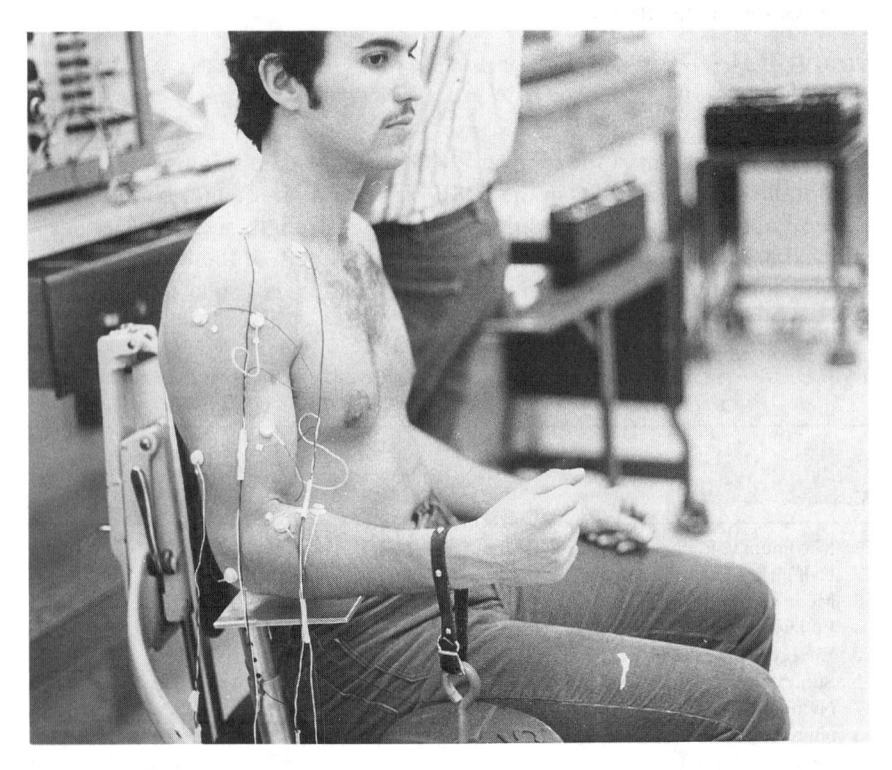

FIGURE 11.20. Multiple site recording of muscle activity has been recommended by Khalil (1973) in order to study the effect of task variables and workplace design on human performance. This method has been referred to as total integrated muscle activity (TIMA).

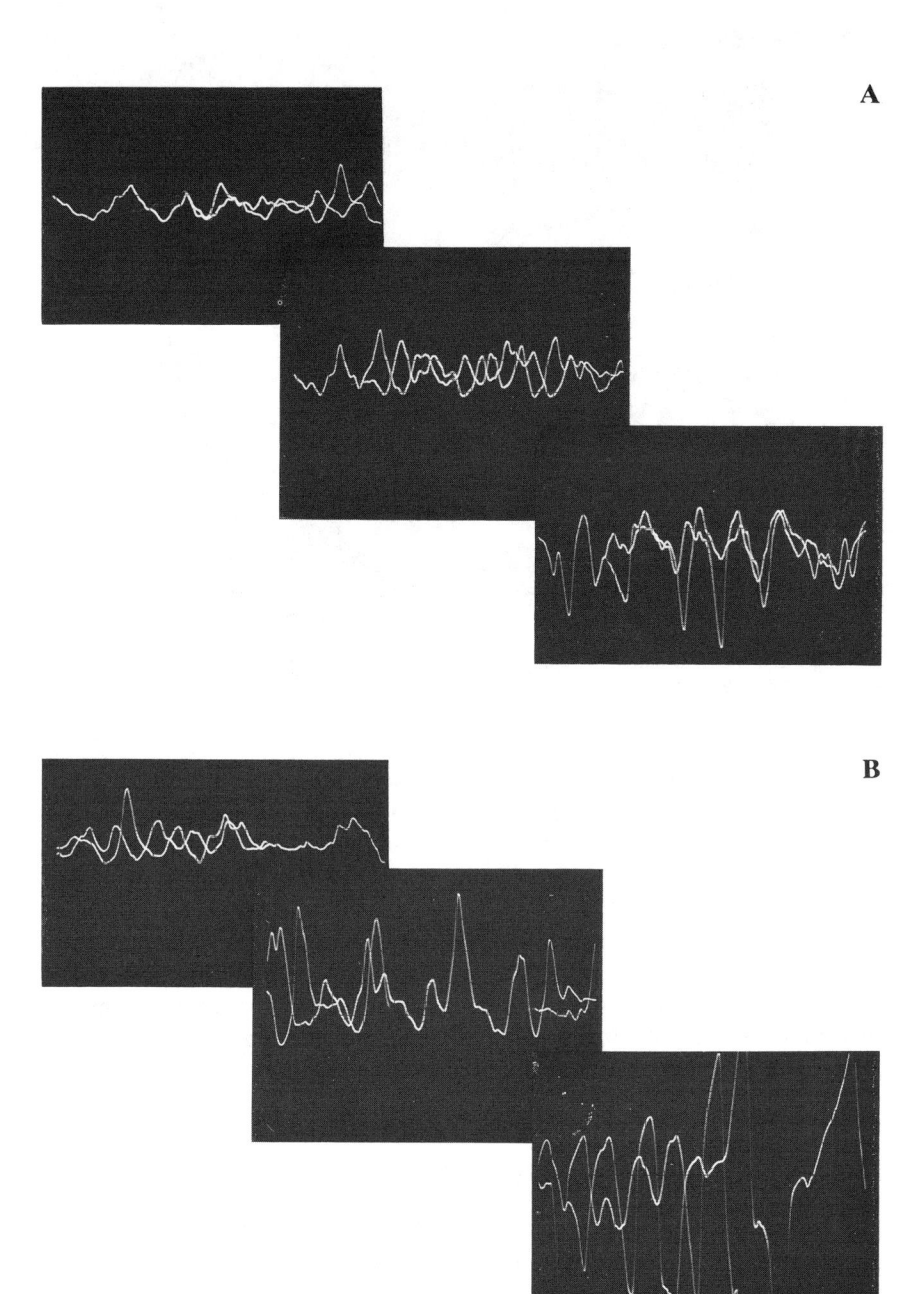

FIGURE 11.21. (A) EMG records corresponding to placing objects at the three bin levels at the beginning of the work cycle. (B) EMG records corresponding to placing objects at the three levels at the end of the work cycle.

179

180   Ergonomics in Back Pain

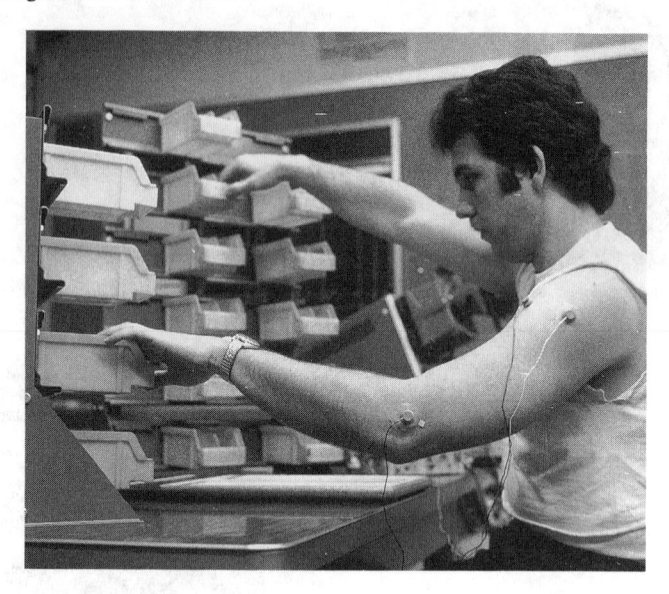

FIGURE 11.22. EMG activity is being recorded while subject is placing objects in bins at various heights (levels).

demonstrate the results of analyzing a task of placing bins at various levels (Fig. 11.22). Electromyography of the deltoid muscle is done when a subject is working at (1) elbow level bin, (2) third level bin, and (3) fifth level bin. Notice the relative level of myoelectric activity when work is performed at elbow height compared to work performed at an elevated bin heights. Electromyography of the same deltoid muscle is done after completion of 15 minutes of continuous work at the three levels of bins. Look at Figure 11.21B and notice the dramatic increase and change in the myoelectric waveform. Overexertion of the muscle due to repetitive motions combined with non-neutral postures can lead to fatigue and muscle contractures.

CASE 3—EMG and Muscle Response to Unexpected Load

It is known that, while the amount of load handled may cause injury, unknown or sudden unexpected loads can be a major contributing factor to injury onset. Unexpected loading can be found in situations involving slipping, struck by, sudden shifting loads, etc. Differences have been demonstrated between muscle response to expected and unexpected loading (Marras et al., 1987; Khalil, Waly, and Zaki, 1990). In simple terms, a subject's expectation of the amount of load has a significant effect on muscle output (Fig. 11.23). The findings suggest that the central nervous system initiates neural signals in proportion to the magnitude of the load it expects. It is believed that it is not until feedback is given to the CNS that the magnitude of the signal is adjusted appropriately to the magnitude of the load (as shown by the initial high EMG corresponding to a heavy load fol-

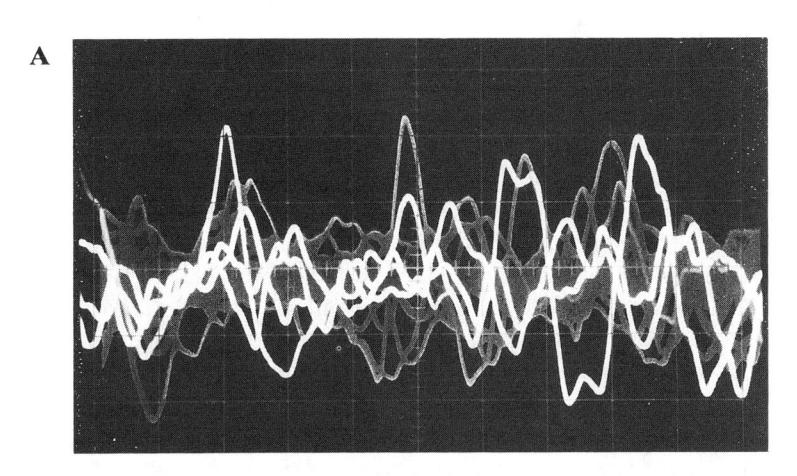

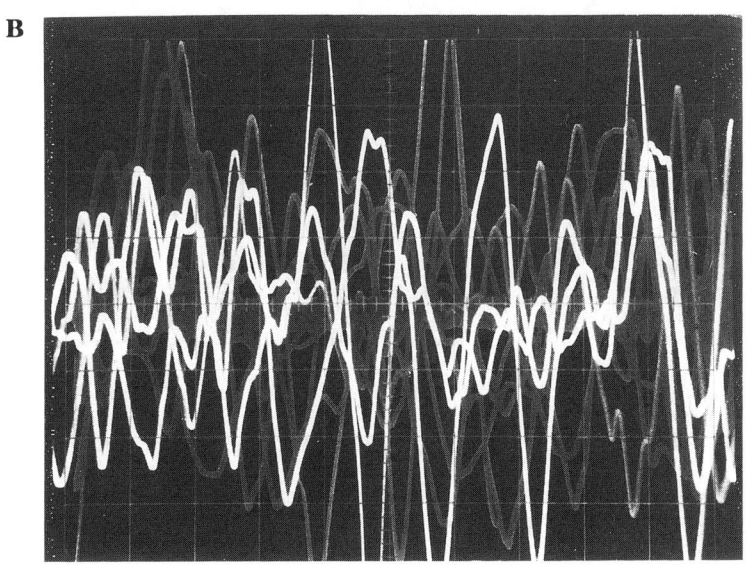

FIGURE 11.23. (A) EMG of a subject expecting to lift 20 pounds and actually lifting 20 lbs. (B) EMG of the same subject expecting to lift 50 lbs. but actually lifting 20 lbs.

182   Ergonomics in Back Pain

lowed by immediate decline of the EMG signal when it was realized that actual load was light). This type of *adjustment* may represent the existence of a *time-lag* between motor signals initiated by the CNS and the adjustment caused by the sensory feedback. This can create a condition of mismatch and imbalance between load demands and muscle work.

PHYSICAL CONDITIONING

CASE 1—Efficacy of FES

Four groups of low back pain patients (40 subjects) and a control group of healthy subjects (10 subjects) participated in a study to compare the efficacy of *passive* and *active* strengthening exercises on the weak quadriceps. The exercise methods were functional electric stimulation (FES) at 20 Hz and 50 Hz, and isometric exercise. Outcome was measured by static strength, limb girth, and electromyographic activity (EMG). Results showed that both methods increased muscle strength over a period of two weeks. However, FES at 20 Hz was more effective in increasing muscle strength than at 50 Hz or isometric exercise. Isometric exercise was more effective in increasing EMG of both the exercised and the contralateral muscles (Fig. 11.24).

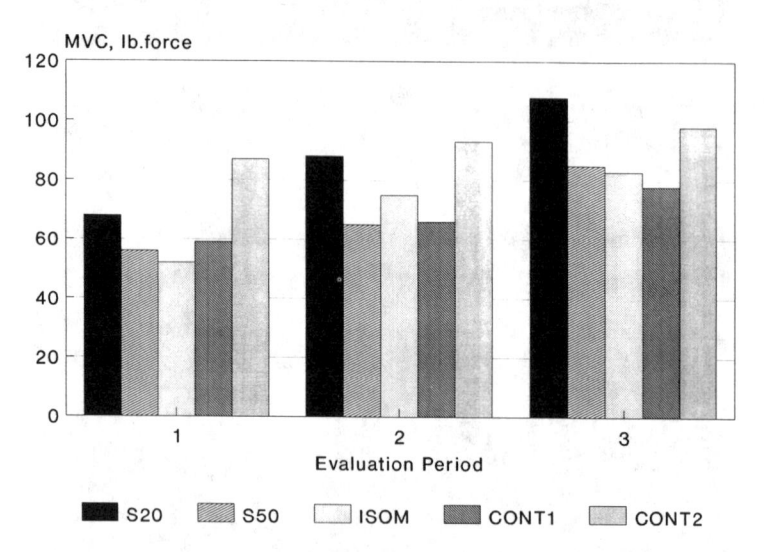

FIGURE 11.24. The effect of FES application on the maximum voluntary contraction force of weak quadriceps muscles in chronic low back pain patients. The effect of FES on increased muscle strength can be seen upon reevaluation (period 2) and at the conclusion of treatment (period 3). In this study there were four groups. Group S20 received stimulation at 20 Hz, and S50 at 50 Hz. Subjects in group ISOM performed isometric exercise. There were two control groups: CONT1 were patients; CONT2 were healthy subjects.

CASE 2—Efficacy of Muscle Reeducation

The efficacy of muscle reeducation (MR) in healthy and low back pain patients was investigated (Khalil, Asfour, Waly, Rosomoff, and Rosomoff, 1987a, b). In this study, 30 patients were assigned to one of two groups: one group underwent the rehabilitation program at the CPRC and the other group participated in the same treatment program in addition to the muscle reeducation modality. Pain level, static strength of back extension, and trunk flexibility (extension and flexion) were the measures of outcome. The results obtained for both groups are summarized in Table 11.7. Results show that all patients exhibited significant improvement in strength and flexibility in only eight days of treatment. The use of the muscle reeducation protocol enhanced the strength and mobility gains. The results of the study prompted implementation of the protocol into clinical practice (Fig. 11.25).

CASE 4—EMG for Evaluating Effects of Stretching

Stretching, mobilization, and manipulation are some of the common techniques used by physical therapists and chiropractors in the rehabilitation of low back pain patients. The effects of these techniques on muscle reconditioning and restoration of muscular function in CLBP patients is not well documented in the medical literature (Quebec Study, 1987).

In a study to quantify the immediate and long-term effects of stretching in the treatment of LBP (Khalil, Asfour et al., 1992), two groups of pa-

TABLE 11.7 Initial and Final Measures of Trunk Function (Khalil, Asfour, Waly, Rosomoff and Rosomoff, 1987a, b)

Group	Variable	Initial Mean	Initial SD	8-Day follow-up Mean	8-Day follow-up SD
Muscle Reeducation					
	Pain Level	6.1	2.9	4.7	2.6
	Strength	50.5	47.0	91.7	52.1
	Flexion ROM	85.3	34.9	125.3	20.8
	Extension ROM	18.4	8.0	30.9	12.8
No Muscle Reeducation					
	Pain Level	5.6	2.4	5.6	2.4
	Strength	63.9	31.9	74.5	44.9
	Flexion ROM	85.5	23.2	119.2	24.3
	Extension ROM	21.3	7.7	30.4	8.8

184   Ergonomics in Back Pain

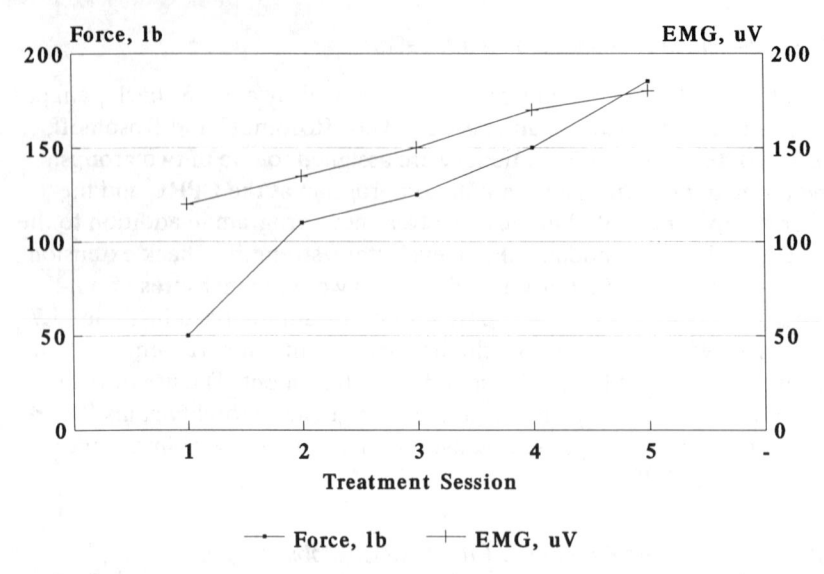

FIGURE 11.25. Changes in lumbar paraspinal EMG activity and isometric trunk extension strength for a 22-year-old male upon muscle reeducation.

tients were studied: a stretching group and a control group. The stretching group received the treatment program at the CPRC plus an added-on systematic stretching program for two weeks (Fig. 11.26). The second group participated in the same treatment program at the CPRC, with the exception that they did not undergo the additional systematic schedule of

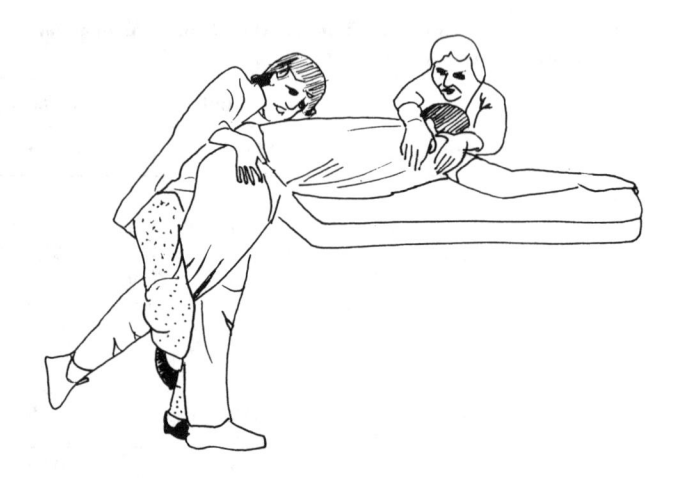

FIGURE 11.26. Illustration of a two-therapist stretching technique.

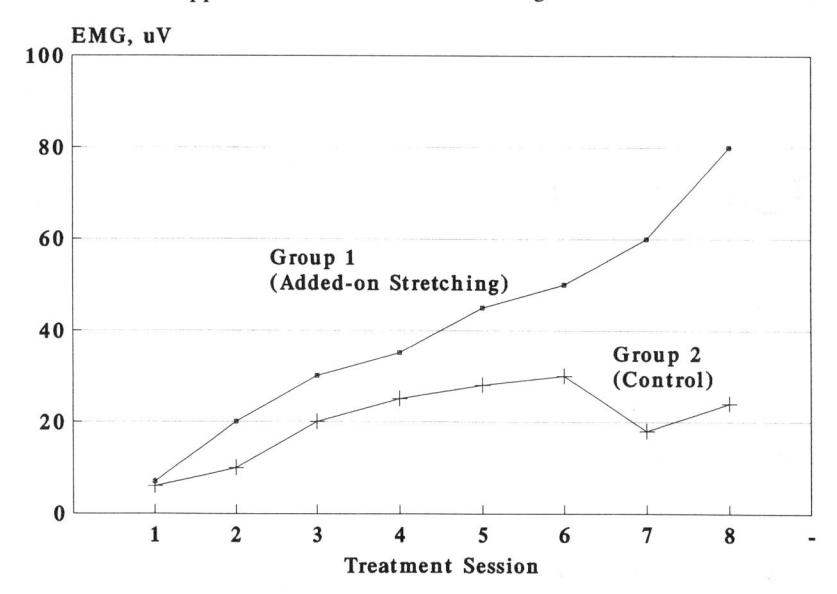

```
         EMG, uV
    100 ┌─────────────────────────────────────┐
        │                                     │
     80 │                                   • │
        │                                     │
        │                                     │
     60 │                               •     │
        │         Group 1                     │
        │      (Added-on Stretching)          │
     40 │                        •            │
        │                   •         Group 2 │
        │              •          +  (Control)│
     20 │         •         +   +             │
        │    +                        +       │
        │ •                                   │
      0 └─────────────────────────────────────┘
          1   2   3   4   5   6   7   8
                  Treatment Session
```

FIGURE 11.27. Effect of introducing an added-on systematic stretching regimen to the rehabilitation program on EMG muscle output of patients in the experimental group and the corresponding changes for the control group.

stretching. The nonsystematic stretching was an integral component of the rehabilitation program for all patients. In order to quantify the effects of the added-on stretching treatment, self-report of pain level (0 to 10), static strength of back extension using the pulling test, lumbar paraspinal muscle activity, trunk and leg flexibility were measured. Patients from both groups in the study were able to improve their functional abilities, as was seen from the significant increase in the static strength of the back extensors and back muscle EMG output. Also, for the two groups, a significant decrease in pain level was found after two weeks of continuous treatment. The use of stretching in a systematic fashion enhanced the functional gains of the LBP patients in the stretching group (Fig. 11.27). There was a significant increase in back muscle EMG, strength, trunk flexion and extension ranges of motion, and straight leg raising; there was significant reduction in pain level for the stretching group over and above what was attained for the control group. These results are in agreement with the generally accepted, but seldomly quantified, notion that stretching has a positive therapeutic effect. Despite the quantification of improvement here, the degree of stretching and its duration remain a subjective criteria dependent on the therapist's experience.

References

Abdel-Moty, A.R., 1992. Stated Versus Observed Performance Levels in Chronic Low Back Pain Patients. Unpublished master thesis, Florida International University, Miami, FL.
Abdel-Moty, E. 1988. "Effects of Functional Electric Stimulation on the Neuromuscular System." Unpublished doctoral dissertation, University of Miami, Coral Gables, FL.
———. 1991. "Functional Capacity Assessment: A Multipurpose Tool." *Back Pain Monitor*, March, pp. 46–48.
Abdel-Moty, E.; Diaz, E.; Khalil, T.M.; Abou Elseoud, M.; Steele-Rosomoff, R.; Rosomoff, H.L. 1992. "Ergonomic Job Analysis for Patients with Cervical Trauma During Rehabilitation." In *Advances in Industrial Ergonomics and Safety*, vol. IV. Edited by S. Kumar. London: Taylor & Francis, pp. 1195–1200.
Abdel-Moty, E.; Field, E.; Miles, N.; and Perez, E. 1991. "Center of Pressure Reproducibility of Comfortable and Predetermined Stances in Healthy Subjects." *Phys Ther* 71:6(suppl):S54.
Abdel-Moty, E.; and Khalil, T.M., 1986a. "Computer-aided Design of the Sitting Workplace." Proceedings of the 8th Annual Conference on Computers and Industrial Engineering, Orlando, FL, pp. 22–26.
———. 1986b. "Computer-aided Design of the Sitting Workplace." *Comput Indust Eng* 11:1–4(suppl):23–26.
———. 1987a. "A Computerized Expert System for Work Simplification and Workplace Design." Proceedings of the Annual International Meeting of Institute of Industrial Engineers, Washington, DC, May 17–21, pp. 665–670.
———. 1987b. "Microcomputers in the Design and Analysis of the VDT Sitting Workplace." In *Trends in Ergonomics/Human Factors, Part A*. Edited by S.S. Asfour. North Holland, Amsterdam: Elsevier Science Publishing B.V., pp. 113–120.
———. 1988a. "Effects of Mechanical Vibration on Peripheral Body Temperature and the Heat Emission Pattern of the Hand." In *Trends in Ergonomics/Human Factors V*. Edited by F. Aghazedh. North-Holland, Amsterdam: Elsevier Science Publishers B.V., pp. 513–519.
———. 1988b. "Computer-Aided Design of the Sitting Workplace: An Expert System

Approach." In *Current Advances in Mechanical Design and Production.* Edited by Y.A. Kabil and M.E. Said. New York: Pergamon Press, pp. 353–360.

———. 1988c. "A Computerized Expert System for Work Simplification and Workplace Design." In *Expert Systems.* Edited by N.A. Botton and T. Raz. Industrial Engineering and Management Press, pp. 221–226.

———. 1988d. "Ergonomics Considerations for the Reduction of Physical Task Demands of Low Back Pain Patients." In *Trends in Ergonomics/Human Factors,* vol. IV. Edited by F. Afaghazedh. North Holland, Amsterdam: Elsevier Science Publishers B.V., pp. 959–967.

———. 1989. "Computer-aided Design of the Sitting Workplace for the Disabled." In *Advances in Ergonomics and Safety I,* Edited by A. Mital. New York: Taylor & Francis, pp. 863–870.

———. 1991. "Computer-aided Design and Analysis of the Sitting workplace for the Disabled." *Int Disab Studies* 13:4:121–124.

Abdel-Moty, E., Khalil, T.M., Asfour, S.; Goldberg, M.,; Rosomoff, R.; and Rosomoff, H. 1990. "On the Relationship Between Age and Responsiveness to Rehabilitation." In *Advances in Industrial Ergonomics and Safety, II.* Edited by B. Das. London: Taylor & Francis, pp. 49–56.

Abdel-Moty, E., Khalil, T.M.; Asfour, S.S.; Howard, M.; Rosomoff, R.S.; and Rosomoff, H.L. 1989. "Effects of Pain on Psychomotor Abilities." In *Advances in Ergonomics and Safety I,* Edited by A. Mital. New York: Taylor & Francis, pp. 465–471.

Abdel-Moty, E.; Khalil, T.M.; Asfour, S.S.; Rosomoff, R.S.; and Rosomoff, H.L. 1988. "Correlation Analysis of the Ergonomics AME: A Method of Defining Patients Progress in a Low Back Pain Rehabilitation Program." Proceedings of the 21st Annual Meeting of the Human Factors Association of Canada /ACE, September 14–16, pp. 65–67.

———. 1988b. "Functional Electrical Stimulation for the Restoration of Muscle Function in Low Back Pain Patients." *Pain Management,* Nov/Dec, 258–263.

———. 1988c. "Ergonomics Considerations for the Reduction of Physical Task Demands of Low Back Pain Patients." In *Trends in Ergonomics/Human Factors,* vol. V. Edited by F. Aghazadeh. Amsterdam, North-Holland Elsevier Science Publishers B.V., pp. 959–967.

Abdel-Moty, E.; Khalil, T.M.; Asfour, S.S.; Sadek, S.; Rosomoff, R.S.; and Rosomoff, H.L. 1991. "Worker's Compensation and Non-Worker's Compensation Chronic Pain Patients Responsiveness to Rehabilitation." *Advances in Industrial Ergonomics & Safety,* III. Edited by W. Karwowski and J.W. Yates. London: Taylor & Francis, pp. 467–474.

Abdel-Moty, E.; Khalil, T.; Diaz, E.; Sadek, S.; Rosomoff, R.; and Rosomoff, H. 1991. "Ergonomic Job Analysis for Patients with Chronic Low Back Pain During Rehabilitation." In *Designing for Everyone.* Edited by Y. Queinnec and F. Daniellou. London: Taylor & Francis, pp. 1638–1640.

Abdel-Moty, E.; Khalil, T.; Fishbain, D.; Asfour, S.; Zaki, A.; Diaz, E.; Sadek, S.; Rosomoff, R.S.; and Rosomoff, H.L. 1991. "Age/Gender Factors and Outcome of Back Pain Rehabilitation." Abstracts of the 10th Annual Scientific Meeting of the American Pain Society, New Orleans, LA, November, p. 119.

Abdel-Moty, E.; Khalil, T.M.; Fishbain, D.; Rosomoff, R.S.; and Rosomoff, H.L. 1991. "Functional Capacity Assessment of Low Back Pain Patients." *Advances in Industrial Ergonomics & Safety,* vol. III. Edited by W. Karwowski and J.W. Yates. London: Taylor & Francis, pp. 475–482.

Abdel-Moty, E.; Khalil, T.; Goldberg, M.; Asfour, S.; Eckstein, E.; and Rosomoff, H. 1990a. "Functional Electric Stimulation (FES) versus Regular Isometric Exercises in the Rehabilitation of Chronic Low Back Pain Patients (CLBPP) with Quadriceps Muscular Weakness." Abstracts of the Annual Meeting of the International Society for the Study of the Lumbar Spine, Boston, MA, June 13–17, p. 43.

Abdel-Moty, E.; Khalil, T.; Goldberg, M.; Rosomoff, R.; and Rosomoff, H. 1990. "Posture and Pain: Health Effects and Ergonomics Interventions." In *Advances in Industrial Ergonomics and Safety*, vol. II. Edited by B. Das. London Taylor & Francis, pp. 117–124.

Abdel-Moty, E.; Khalil, T.M.; Rosomoff, R.S.; and Rosomoff, H.L., 1987. "Computerized Electromyography in Quantifying the Effectiveness of Functional Electrical Stimulation." In *Trends in Ergonomics/Human Factors*, vol. IV-A, Edited by S.S. Asfour. New-Holland, Amsterdam: Elsevier Science Publishers B.V., pp. 1057–1065.

———. 1990. "Ergonomics Considerations and Interventions." In *Painful Cervical Trauma: Diagnosis and Rehabilitative Treatment of Neuromusculoskeletal Injuries.* Edited by C.D. Tollison and J.R. Satterthwaite. Baltimore, Maryland: Williams & Wilkins, pp. 214–229.

Abdel-Moty, E.; Khalil, T.M.; Sadek, S.; Dilsen, E.K.; Fishbain, D.; Steele-Rosomoff, R.; and Rosomoff, H.L. 1992. "Functional Capacity Assessment: A Test Battery and Its Use in Rehabilitation." In *Advances in Industrial Ergonomics and Safety,* vol. IV. Edited by S. Kumar. London: Taylor & Francis, pp. 1171–1178.

Addison R.; and Schultz A. 1980. "Trunk Strengths in Patients Seeking Hospitalization for Chronic Low Back Disorders." *Spine* 5:6:539–544.

Agarwal G.G. 1975. "An Analysis of the EMG by Fourier: Simulation and Experimental Techniques." *IEEE Trans Biomed Eng* BME-22:225–229.

Alfieri, V. 1982. "Electrical Treatment of Spasticity: Reflex Tonic Activity in Hemiplegic Patients and Selected Specific Electrostimulation." *Scand J Rehab Med.* 14:4:177–182.

Alston, W.; Carlson, K.E.; Feldman, D.J.; Grimm, Z.; and Gerontinos, E. 1966. "A Quantitative Study of Muscle Factors in the Chronic Low Back Syndrome." *J Am Geriat Soc* 14:1041–1047.

American College of Sports Medicine. 1976. "Guidelines for Graded Exercise Testing and Prescription," 3rd ed. Philadelphia: Lea & Febiger.

American Medical Association. 1988. "Guides to the Evaluation of Permanent Impairment." Edited by Alan L. Engelberg. Chicago: American Medical Association.

———. 1990. "Guides to the Evaluation of Permanent Impairment," 3rd ed. (revised). Chicago: American Medical Association.

Anderson, C.K.; Chaffin, D.B.; Herrin, G.D.; and Mathews, L.S. 1985. "A Biomechanical Model of the Lumbar Joint During Lifting Activities." *J Biomech* 18:571–584.

Andersson, G.B.J.; Chaffin, D.B.; and Pope, M.H. 1984. "Occupational Biomechanics of the Lumbar Spine." In *Occupational Low Back Pain*. Edited by Pope, M.H., Frymoyer, J.W., and Andersson, G.B.J. New York: Praeger, pp. 39–70.

Andersson, G.B.J.; Schultz, A.B.; and Ortengren, R. 1986. "Trunk Muscle Forces During Desk Work." *Ergonomics* 29:9:1113–1127.

ANSI. 1988. "American National Standard for Human Factors Engineering of VDT Workstations." Santa Monica: Human Factors Society.

Ariel, G.B. 1983. "Resistive Training." *Clinics Sports Med* 2:1:55–69.

Ariel Performance Analysis System. Computerized Biomechanical Analysis, Inc. 22000 Plano Trabuco Road, Trabuco Canyon, CA 92678.

Armstrong, J.R. 1965. *Lumbar Disc Lesions*. Baltimore: Williams & Wilkins.

Asfour, S.S.; Ayoub, M.M.; and Genaidy, A.M. 1984. "A Psychophysical Study of the Effect of Task Variables on Lifting and Lowering Tasks." *J Human Ergology* 13:3–14.

Asfour, S.S.; Ayoub, M.M.; Genaidy, A.M.; and Khalil, T.M. 1986. "A Database of Physiological Responses to Manual Lifting." In *Trends in Ergonomics/Human Factors*, III Part B, Edited by W. Karawowski. North Holland, Amsterdam: Elsevier Publishers B.V., pp. 801–809.

Asfour, S.; Ayoub, M.M.; and Mital, A. 1984. "Effects of an Endurance and Strength Training Programme on Lifting Capability of Males." *Ergonomics*, 27:4:435–442.

Asfour, S.S., Dutta, S.P., and Taboun, S.M. 1984. "The Effects of Training on Static Strength and Carrying Capacity of College Males." In *Trends in Ergonomics/Human Factors*, I, Edited by A. Mital. Netherlands: Amsterdam Elsevier Science Publishers B.V.

Asfour, S.S.; Genaidy, A.M.; and Khalil, T.M. 1987. "An On-line Microcomputer-based Metabolic Monitoring System." *Int J Indust Ergonomics*, 1:3:169–177.

———. 1985. "The Relationship Between Frequency of Lift and Lifting Capacity." In *Ergonomics International*. I.O. Brown, R. Goldsmith, K. Coombes, and M.A. Sinclair. London: Taylor & Francis, pp. 865–867.

Asfour, S.S.; Genaidy, A.M.; Khalil, T.M.; and Greco, E.C. 1984. "Physiological and Pychophysical Determination of Lifting Capacity for Low Frequency Lifting Tasks." In *Trends in Ergonomics/Human Factors*, vol. I. Edited by A. Mital. North Holland, Amsterdam: Elsevier Science Publishers B.V., pp. 149–153.

———. 1985. "A Combined Approach for Determination of Lifting Capacity." In *Trends in Ergonomics/Human Factors*, vol. II, Edited by R.E. Eberts and C.G. Eberts. North Holland, Amsterdam: Elsevier Science Publishers B.V., pp. 617–623.

Asfour, S.S.; Genaidy, A.M.; and Khalil, T.M.; Muthuswamy, S. 1986a. "Physiologic Responses to Static, Dynamic, and Combined Tasks." *Am Indust Hyg Assoc J* 47:12:798–802.

———. 1986b. "An On-line Microcomputer-based Respiratory Monitor for Manual Materials Handling." *Comput Indust Eng*, 11:1–4:146–150.

Asfour, S.S.; Khalil, T.M.; Moty, E.A.; Steele, R., and Rosomoff, H.L. 1983. "Low Back Pain: A Challenge to Productivity." Proceedings of 7th Industrial Engineering Conference. Windsor, Canada, pp. 813–818.

Asfour, S.S.; Khalil, T.M.; Waly, S.M.; Goldberg, M.L.; Rosomoff, R.S.; and Rosomoff, H.L. 1990. "Biofeedback in Back Muscle Strengthening." *Spine* 15:6:510–513.

Astrand, P.O. 1960. "Aerobic Work Capacity in Men and Women with Special Reference to Age." *Acta Physiol Scand* 49 (suppl), p. 169.

———. 1976. "Quantification of Exercise Capability and Evaluation of Physical Capacity in Man." *Cardiovasc Dis* 19:51.

Ayoub, M.M. 1977. "Optimum Design of Containers for Manual Materials Handling Tasks." *Appl Ergonomics* 8:67–72.

Ayoub, M.M.; Bethea, N.J.; Deivanayagau, S.; Asfour, S.S.; Bakken, G.M.; Liles, E.; Mital, A.; and Sherif, M. 1978. "Determination and Modelling of Lifting Capacity." Final Report, DHEW (NIOSH) Grant 5 R01 OH 00545-02.

Ayoub, M.M., and El-Bassoussi, M.M. 1978. "Dynamic Biomechanical Model for Saggital Plan Lifting Activities." In *Safety in Manual Materials Handling*. Edited by C.G. Drury. DHEW (NIOSH) Publication No. 78–185, pp. 120–130.

Balke, B.; and Ware, R.W. 1971. "An Experimental Study of Physical Fitness of Air Force Personnel." *U.S. Armed Forces Med J* 10:675.

Bandura, A. 1977. "Self-efficacy: Toward a Unifying Theory of Behavioral Change." *Psychology Rev* 84, 191–215.

Bandura, A. 1986. *Social Foundations of Thoughts and Action*. Englewood Cliffs, New Jersey: Prentice Hall.

Barnes, D.; and Benjamin, S. 1987. "The Self Care Assessment Schedule" (SCAS). *J Psychosomatic Res* 31, 191–202.

Barnes, R.M. 1988. *Motion and Time Study Design and Measurement of Work*. New York: John Wiley & Sons.

Basmajian, J.V. 1979. *Muscles Alive: Their Function Revealed by Electromyography*, 4th ed. Baltimore: Williams & Wilkins.

Basmajian, J.V.; Clifford, H.C.; McLeod, W.D., 1975. *Computers in Electromyography*. London: Butterworth.

Basmajian, J.V.; and DeLuca, C.J. 1985. *Muscles Alive*. Baltimore: Williams & Wilkins.

Battie, M.C.; Bigos, S.J.; Fisher, L.D.; Hansson, T.H.; Jones, M.E.; and Wortley, M.D. 1989. "Isometric Lifting Strength as a Predictor of Industrial Back Pain Reports." *Spine* 14:8:851–856.

Battista, M.E. 1990. "Disability Evaluations: Expectations of Insurers and Payors." *J Disab* 1:3:168–177.

Bergmans, J. 1973. "Computer-assisted Measurement of the Parameters of Single Motor Potentials in Human Electromyography." In *New Development in Electromyography and Clinical Neurophysiology,* vol. 2, Edited by J.E. Desmedt. Karger, Basel: pp. 482–488.

Bergquist-Ulman, M.; and Larsson, U. 1977. "Acute Low Back Pain in Industry: A Controlled Prospective Study with Special Reference to Therapy and Confounding Factors." *Acta Orthop Scand* 170(suppl).:1–117.

Beruvides, M.G.; and Khalil, T.M. 1984. "VDT Ergonomics: A Survey and Guidelines." Proceeding of the Fall Industrial Engineering Conference, pp. 357–364.

Berzuini, C.; Maranzana-Figini, M.; and Bernadinelli, L. 1982. "Effective Use of EMG Parameters in the Assessement of Neuromuscular Diseases." *Int'l J Biomed Comput* 3:481–499.

Biering-Sorensen, F. 1984. "Physical Measurements as Risk Indicators of Low Back Trouble Over a One-year Period." *Spine* 9:106–119.

Bigland-Ritchie, B. 1981. "EMG/Force Relations and Fatigue of Human Voluntary Contractions." *Exer Sports Sci Rev* 9:75–117.
Bohannon, R.W. 1983. "Effect of Electrical Stimulation to the Vastus Medialis Muscle in a Patient with Chronically Dislocating Patella." *Phys Ther* 63:9:1445–1447.
Bond, M.B. 1970. "Low Back Injuries in Industry." *Ind Med* 39:5:28–32.
Bonica, J.J. 1953. *The Management of Pain*. Philadelphia: Lea & Febiger.
Bonica, J. 1980. "Pain Research and Therapy: Past and Current Status and Future Needs." In *Pain, Discomfort, Humanitarian Care in Developments in Neurology*. Edited by J. Bonica, L. Ng. North Holland, Amsterdam: Elsevier Science Publishers B.V. pp. 1–46.
———. 1981. "A Review of Multidisciplinary Pain Clinics and Pain Centers." *NIDA Res Monog* 36:VII–X.
———. 1988. "Evolution of Multidisciplinary/Interdisciplinary Pain Programs." In *Pain Centers: A Revolution in Health Care*. Edited by G.M. Aronoff. New York: Raven Press, pp. 9–32.
Brena, S.F.; and Turk, D.C. 1988. "Vocational Disability: A Challenge to Pain Rehabilitation Programs." In *Pain Centers—A Revolution in Health Care*. Edited by G.M. Arnoff. New York. Raven Press, pp. 167–180.
Brouha, L. 1960. *Physiology in Industry*. New York: Pergamon Press.
Brunarski, D.J. 1984. "Clinical Trials of Spinal Manipulation: A Critical Appraisal and Review of the Literature." *J Manipulative Physiol Ther* 7:243–249.
Business & Health. 1990. Published by American Health Consultants, Inc., p. 8.
Cady, L.D.; Bischoff, D.P.; O'Connell, E.R.; Thomas, P.C.; and Allan, J.H. 1979. "Strength and Fitness and Subsequent Back Injuries in Firefighters." *J Occup Med* 21:269–272.
Cailliet, R. 1980. *Soft Tissue Pain and Disability*. Philadelphia: F.A. Davis.
———. 1981. *Low Back Syndrome*. Philadelphia: F.A. Davis.
Carbines, M.E. and Schawrtz, G.E. 1987. *Strategies for Managing Disability Costs*. A Publication of the Washington Business Group on Health/Institute for Rehabilitation and Disability Management, p. 1.
Carr, D.B.; Bullen, B.A.; Skrinar, G.S. 1981. "Physical Conditioning Facilitates the Exercise-induced Secretion of Beta Endorphine and Beta-hypoprotein in Women." *N Eng J Med* 305:560–563.
Cassisi, J.E.; Sypert, G.W.; Solomon, A.; and Kapel, L. 1989. "Independent Evaluation of a Multidisciplinary Rehabilitation Program for Chronic Low Back Pain." *Neurosurgery* 25:6:877–883.
Chaffin, D.B. 1969a. "Electromyography–A Method of Measuring Local Muscle Fatigue." *J Methods-Time Measur* 14:2:29–36.
———. 1969b. "A Computerized Biomechanical Model Development of and Use in Studying Gross Body Actions." *J Biomech* 2:429–441.
———. 1974. "Human Strength Capability and Low Back Pain." *J Occup Med*, 16:248–254.
———. 1975. "Ergonomics Guide for the Assessment of Human Strength." *Am Indust Hyg Assoc J* 36:505–510.
Chaffin, D.B.; and Andersson, G.B.J. 1984. *Occupational Biomechanics*. New York: John Wiley & Sons.

Chaffin, D.B., Herrin, G.D., and Keyserling, M.S., 1978. "Pre-employment Strength Testing: An Update Position." *J Occup Med* 20:403–408.

Clapper, M.P.; and Wolf, S.L. 1988. "Comparison of the Reliability of the Orthoranger and the Standard Goniometer for Assessing Active Lower Extremity Range of Motion." *Phys Ther*, 68:214–218.

Council, J.R.; Ahren, D.K.; Follick, M.J; and Kline, C.L. 1988. "Expectancies and Functional Impairment in Chronic Low Back Pain." *Pain* 33:323–331.

Culter, B.; Fishbain, D.; Goldberg, M.; Abdel-Moty, E.; Steele-Rosomoff, R.; and Rosomoff, H. 1991. "Psychiatric Dual Diagnosis/Co-morbidity in Chronic Pain Patients Who Misuse Drugs." Abstracts of the American Pain Society Meeting. November 7–10, New Orleans, LA, p. 131.

Currier, D.P., Mann, R. 1983. "Muscular Strength Development by Electrical Stimulation in Healthy Individuals." *Phys Ther* 63:6:915–921.

Cypress, B.K. 1983. "Characteristics of Physician Visits for Back Symptoms: A National Perspective." *Am J Public Health* 73:389–395.

Damkot, D.K.; Pope, M.H. 1982. "The Relationship Between Work History, Work Environment and Low Back Pain in Males." *Spine* 9:4:395–399.

Dehlin, O.; Hedenrud, B.; and Horal, J. 1976. "Back Symptoms in Nursing Aids in a Geriatric Hospital." *Scand J Rehab Med* 8:47.

Deyo, R.A.; and Tsui-Wu, Y.J.; 1987. Descriptive Epidemiology of Low Back Pain and Its Related Medical Care in the United States. *Spine* 12:3:265–268.

Diaz, E.; Khalil, T.; Asfour, S.; and Abdel-Moty, E. 1991. "Integration of Ergonomics and Product Design: A Computerized Database System." In *Designing for Everyone*. Edited by Y. Queinnec and F. Daniellou. London: Taylor & Francis, pp. 1049–1051.

Dolce, J.J.; Crocker, M.F.; and Dolys, D.M. 1986. "Prediction of Outcome Among Chronic Pain Patients." *Behav Res Ther* 24:313–319.

Drury, C.G.; Francher, M. 1985. "Evaluation of Forward Sloping Chair." *Applied Ergonomics*, pp. 41–47

Emmanuel, I.; Chafee, J.; and Wing, J. 1956. A Study of Human Weight Lifting Capabilities for Loading Ammunition into the F-86 Aircraft. U.S. Air Force, WADC-TR 056-367.

Esser, G. 1983. Overview of Vocational Evaluation. Stout University Training Workshop, Las Vegas, NV.

Fairbank, J.C.; O'Brien, J.P.; and Davis, P.R. 1980. "Intraabdominal Pressure Rise During Weight Lifting as an Objective Measure of Low Back Pain." *Spine* 5:179–184.

Fairbank, J.C.T.; Pynsent, P.B.; Van Poortvliet, J.A.; and Phillips, H. 1984. "Influence of Anthropometric Factors and Joint Laxity on the Incidence of Adolescent Back Pain." *Spine* 9:461–464.

Ferreira, S.H. 1983. "Prostaglandins: Peripheral and Central Analgesia." In *Advances in Pain Research and Therapy*, vol V. Edited by J.J. Bonica, New York: Raven Press, p. 597.

Field, E.; Abdel-Moty, E.; Khalil, T.; and Asfour, S. 1991. "Postural Proprioception in Healthy and Back Injured Adults." *Phys Ther* 71:6(suppl):S104.

Fish, D.R.; Wingate, L. 1985. "Sources of Goniometric Error at the Elbow." *Phys Ther* 65:1666–1670.

Fishbain, D.A.; Abdel-Moty, E.; Cutler, R.; Khalil, T.M.; Rosomoff, R.S.; and Rosomoff, H.L. 1992. A Method of Measuring Residual Functional Capacity in Chronic Pain Patients. Submitted for publication.

Fishbain, D.; Cutler, B.; Abdel-Moty, E.; Steele-Rosomoff, R.; and Rosomoff, H. 1991. "Patient Self-Rated Outcome of Pain Center Treatment Measured by Rating Scale." Abstracts of the American Pain Society Meeting, New Orleans, LA, November 7–10, p. 112.

Fishbain, D.A.; Goldberg, M.L.; Khalil, T.M.; Santana, R.; Rosomoff, H.L.; Abdel-Moty, E. 1988. "The Utility of Electromyographic Feedback in the Treatment of Conversion Paralysis." *Am J Psych* 145:12:1572–1575.

Fishbain, D.A.; Goldberg, M.; Labbe, E.; 1988. "Compensation and Non-compensation Chronic Pain Patients Compared for DSM-III Operational Diagnoses." *Pain* 32:197–206.

Fishbain, D.A.; Goldberg, M.; Meagher, B.R.; Steele, R., and Rosomoff, H. 1986. "Male and Female Chronic Pain Patients Categorized by DSM-III Psychiatric Diagnostic Criteria." *Pain* 26:181–197.

Fishbain, D.; Goldberg, M.; Rosomoff, H.; Steele-Rosomoff, R.; Jorge, M.; and Abdel-Moty, E. 1991a. "Chronic Pain and Suicide Death." Abstracts of the 144th Annual Meeting of the American Psychiatric Association, New Orleans, LA, May 11–16, p. 177.

———. 1991b. "Clonazepam Open Clinical Trial for Chronic Pain of Myofascial Pain Syndrome Origin Refractory to Pain Treatment." Abstracts of the 144th Annual Meeting of the American Psychiatric Association, New Orleans, LA, May 11–16, p. 177.

Fishbain, D.A.; Goldberg, M.; Steele, R.; and Rosomoff, H. 1989. "DSM-III Diagnoses of Patients with Myofascial Pain Syndrome (Fibrositis)." *Arch Phys Med Rehab* 70:6:433–438.

Fishbain, D.A.; and Rosomoff, H.L. 1987. "Myofascial Pain Syndrome." *Pain* 29:265–266.

Fishbain, D.; Rosomoff, R.S.; Goldberg, M.L.; Jorge, M.; Zaki, T.M.; Abdel-Moty, E.; and Khalil, T. 1990. "Magnesium Levels in Chronic Pain Patients." *Clin J Pain* 7:1:61.

Fortune, 1992. "Let's Really Cure the Health System." March 23, p. 46.

Frymoyer, J.W. 1988. "Back Pain and Sciatica." *N Engl J Med* 318:291–300.

Frymoyer, J.W.; Pope, M.H.; Clements, J. 1983. "Risk Factors in Low Back Pain." *J Bone Joint Surg* 65A:213–218.

Garg, A. and Chaffin, D.B. 1975. "A Biomechanical Computerized Simulation of Human Strength." *Am Instit Indust Eng Trans* 7:1–15.

Gerber, A.; Studer, R.M.; Figueiredo, R.P.; and Moschytz, G.S. 1984. "A New Framework and Computer Program for Quantitative EMG Signal Analysis." *IEEE Trans Biomed Eng* 31:12:857–863.

Godfrey, C.M.; Jayawardena, H.; Quance, T.A.; and Welsh, P. 1979. "Comparison of Electro-stimulation and Isometric Exercise in Strengthening the Quadriceps Muscle." *Physiotherapy* (Canada), 31:5:265–267.

Gould, N.; Donnermeyer, D.; Pope, M.; and Ashikaga, T. 1982. "Transcutaneous Muscle Stimulation as a Method to Retard Disuse Atrophy." *Clin Orthop* 164:215–220.

Grandjean, E. 1980. *Fitting the Task to the Man—An Ergonomic Approach.* London: Taylor & Francis.

———. 1988. *Fitting the Task to the Man: A Text Book of Occupational Ergonomics,* 4th ed. New York: Taylor & Francis.

Granger, C.V.; and Greer, D.S. 1976. "Functional Status Measurement and Medical Rehabilitation Outcomes." *Arch Phys Med Rehab* 57:103–109.

Granstrom, E. 1983. "Biochemistry of the Prostaglandins, Thromboxanes, and Leukotrienes." In *Advances in Pain Research and Therapy,* vol 5. Edited by J.J. Bonica et al. New York: Raven Press, p. 605.

Greco, E.C.; Khalil, T.M.; and Moty, E.A. 1982. "Vibration Induced Synchronization in Myoelectric Activity." 35th ACEMB Meeting, Philadelphia, PA, p. 197.

Grieve, D.W.; and Cavanagh, P.R. 1973. "The Quantitative Analysis of Phasic Electromyography.' In *New Development in Electromyography and Clinical Neurophysiology* vol 2. Edited by J.E. Desmedt. Basel: Karger, pp. 489–496.

Haber, L.D. 1971. "Disabling Effects of Chronic Disease and Impairment." *J Chronic Dis* 24:469–487.

Hadler, N. 1977. "Industrial Rheumatology: Clinical Investigations into the Influence of the Pattern of Usage on the Pattern of Regional Musculoskeletal Disease." *Arthritis and Rheumatism* 20:1019–1024.

Hadler, N.M. 1978. "Legal Ramification of the Medical Definition of Back Disease." *Ann Intern Med* 89:992–999.

Hagg, G. 1981. "Electromyographic Fatigue Analysis Based on the Number of Zero Crossings." *Pfluger Arch* 391:78–80.

Hall, H.; Iceton, J.A. 1983. "Back School: An Overview with Specific Reference to the Canadian Back Education Units." *Clin Orthop* 179:10–17.

Hannson, T.H.; Stanely, J.B.; Wortley, M.K.; and Spengler, D.M. 1984. "The Load on the Lumbar Spine During Isometric Strength Testing." *Spine* 9:877–884.

Hasue, M.; and Fujiwara, M. 1979. "Epidemiologic and Clinical Studies in Long-Term Prognosis of Low Back Pain and Sciatica." *Spine* 4:150–155.

Hausmanowa-Petrusevicz, I.; and Kopec, J. 1983. "Quantitative EMG and its Automation." In *Computer-Aided Electromyography.* (Prog. Clin. Neurophysiol., Vol. 10), Edited by J.E. Desmedt. Basel: Karger.

Heinrich, H.W. 1959. *Industrial Accident Prevention,* 4th ed. New York:McGraw-Hill.

Herbert, M.A. 1983. "The Treatment of Scoliosis Using Electrical Stimulation." *Eng Med Biol,* Sept. 43–50.

Hirsch, C.; Jonsson, B.; and Lewin, T. 1969. "Low-back Symptoms in Swedish Female Population." *Clin Orthop* 63:171–176

Holmes, D. 1985. "The Role of the Occupational Therapist—Work Evaluator." *Am J Occup Ther* 39:5:308–313.

Holzman, A., Turk, D. 1986. *Pain Management: A Handbook of Psychological Treatment Approaches.* New York: Pergamon Press.

Horal, J. 1969. "The Clinical Appearance of Low Back Disorders in the City of Gothenberg, Sweden." *Acta Orthop Scand.* 118(suppl.):171–176.

Hult, L. 1954. "The Munkfors Investigation." *Acta Orthop Scand* 16(suppl).
———. 1954. "Cervical, Dorsal, and Lumbar Spinal Syndromes." *Acta Orthop Scand* 17(suppl).
Hultman, E.; Sjoholm, V.; and Jaderholm, E.K. 1983. "Evaluation of Methods of Electrical Stimulation of Human Skeletal Muscles in Situ." *Pflugers Arch* 398:139–141.
Hurme, M.; and Alaranta, H. 1987. "Factors Predicting the Result of Surgery for Lumbar Intervertebral Disc Herniation." *Spine* 12:933–937.
IASP Subcommittee on Taxonomy. 1979. "Pain terms: A List with Definitions and Notes on Usage." *Pain* 6:249–252.
Ignelzi, R.J.; Sternback, R.A.; and Timmermans, G. 1977. "The Pain Ward Follow-up Analysis." *Pain* 3:277–285.
Inbar, G.F.; and Noujaim, A.E. 1984. "On Surface EMG Spectral Characterization and Its Application to Diagnostic Classification." *IEEE Trans Biomed Eng* 31:9:597–604.
International Association for the Study of Pain Subcommittee on Taxonomy. 1986. "Classification of chronic pain." *Pain* 3(suppl).
Jackson, K.M. 1982. "Digital Analysis of Electromyograms: A Fortran Package." *Electromyogr Clin Neurophys* 22:65–87.
Jensen, M.P.; Turner, J.A.; and Romano, J.A. 1991. "Self-efficacy and Outcome Expectancies: Relationship to Chronic Pain Coping Strategies and Adjustment." *Pain* 44:263–269.
Jette, A.M. 1980a. "Functional Capacity Evaluation: Empirical Approach." *Arch Phys Med Rehab* 61:85–89.
———. 1980b. "Functional Status Index: Reliability of a Chronic Disease Evaluation Instrument." *Arch Phys Med Rehab* 61:395–401.
Kaiser, E.; and Petersen, I. 1965. "Muscle Action Potentials Studied by Frequency Analysis and Duration Measurement." *Acta Neurol Scand,* 41:19–41.
Katz, S.; Downs, T.D.; Cash, H.R.; and Grotz, R.C. 1970. "Progress in Development of Index of ADL." *Gerontologist* 10, 20–30.
Keim, H.A. 1981. *How to Care for Your Back.* New Jersey: Prentice-Hall.
Kelsey, J.L. 1975. "An Epidemiological Study of Acute Herniated Lumbar Intervertebral Disc." *Rheumatol Rehab* 14:144–159.
Kelsey, J.L.; Pastides, H.; and Bisbee, G.E. 1978. *Musculoskeletal Disorders: Their Frequency of Occurrence and Their Impact on the Population of the United States.* New York: Neale Watson Academic Publications.
Kelsey, J.L.; White, A.A.; Pastides, H.; and Bisbee, G.E. 1979. "The Impact of Musculoskeletal Disorders on the Population of the United States." *J Bone Joint Surg* 61:959–964.
Keyserling W.M. 1982. "Strength Testing as a Method of Evaluating Ability to Perform Strenuous Work." In *Chronic Low Back Pain.* Edited by M. Stanton-Hicks and R. Boas. New York: Raven Press.
Keyserling, W.M.; Herrin, G.D.; and Chaffin, D.B. 1980. "Isometric Strength Testing as a Means of Controlling Medical Incidents on Strenuous Jobs." *J Occup Med* 22:332–336.
Khalil, T.M. 1970. "The Biomechanical Approach to Measuring Human Work."

Proceedings of the Institute of Manag. Science, Winter Symposium, Gainseville, FL.

———. 1972. "Design Tools and Machines to Fit the Man." *Indus Eng* 1:32–35.

———. 1973. "An Electromyographic Methodology for the Evaluation of Industrial Design." *Human Factors* 15:3:257–264.

———. 1974. "Ergonomics—A Growing Domain for Dentistry." *Ergonomics* 17:1:75–86.

———. 1976. "The Role of Ergonomics in Increasing Productivity." Proceedings of the AIIE National Conference, St. Louis, MO.

Khalil, T.M.; Abdel-Moty, E.; Asfour, S.S.; Fishbain, D.A.; Rosomoff, R.S.; and Rosomoff, H.L. 1988. "Functional Electric Stimulation in the Reversal of Conversion Disorder Paralysis." *Arch Phys Med Rehab* 69:7:545–547.

Khalil, T.; Abdel-Moty, E.; Asfour, S.; Fishbain, D.; Sadek, S.; Diaz, E.; Zaki, A.; Rosomoff, R.S.; and Rosomoff, H.L. 1991. "Compensation Status and Outcome of Back Pain Rehabilitation." Abstracts of the 10th Annual Scientific Meeting of the American Pain Society, New Orleans, LA, November, p. 119

Khalil, T.; Abdel-Moty, E.; Asfour, S.; Goldberg, M.; Rosomoff, R.; and Rosomoff, H. 1990. "The Relationship Between Self-Report of Pain Level (SRPL) and Psychophysical Static Lifting Abilities in Chronic Low Back Pain (CLBP) Patients." Abstracts of the Annual Meeting of the International Society for the Study of the Lumbar Spine, Boston, MA, June 13–17, p. 16.

Khalil, T.M.; Abdel-Moty, E.; Asfour, S.S.; Rosomoff, R.S.; and Rosomoff, H.L. 1990. "Ergonomics in the Management of Occupational Injuries." In *Industrial Ergonomics: Case Studies*. Edited by B.M. Pulat and D.C. Alexander. Norcross, Georgia: Industrial Engineering and Management Press, pp. 41–53.

Khalil, T.; Abdel-Moty, E.; Ayoub, M.M.; and Fishbain, D. 1991. "Practical Approaches to Functional Capacity Evaluations of Chronic Low Back Pain Patients." Abstracts of the 10th Annual Scientific Meeting of the American Pain Society, New Orleans, LA, November, p. 30.

Khalil, T.M.; Abdel-Moty, E.; Diaz, E.; Rosomoff, R.S.; and Rosomoff, H.L. 1991. "Electromyographic Symmetry Pattern in Patients with Chronic Low Back Pain and Comparison to Controls." In *Advances in Industrial Ergonomics and Safety*, vol. III. Edited by W. Karwowski and J.W. Yates. Taylor & Francis, Ltd., pp. 483–490.

Khalil, T.; Abdel-Moty, E.; and Fishbain, D. 1990. "Functional Capacity Assessment of Patients with Chronic Low Back Pain." Abstracts of the American Pain Society Annual Meeting, St. Louis, Missouri, p. 102.

Khalil, T.; Abdel-Moty, E.; Goldberg, M.; Rosomoff, R.; and Rosomoff, H. 1990. "Aging and Outcome of Back Pain Rehabilitation." Abstracts of the American Academy of Physical Medicine and Rehabilitation/American Congress of Rehabilitation Medicine Meeting, Phoenix, AZ, p. 117.

Khalil, T.M.; Abdel-Moty, E.; Rosomoff, R.; and Rosomoff, H.L. 1991. "Efficacy of Physical Restoration in the Elderly. Experimental Aging Research." In Print.

Khalil, T.M.; Abdel-Moty, E.; Sadek, S.; Dilsen, E.K.; Steele-Rosomoff, R.; and Rosomoff, H.L. 992. "Postural Sway and Balance in Healthy Subjects and in

Patients with Chronic Pain." In: *Advances in Industrial Ergonomics and Safety*, vol. IV. Edited by S. Kumar. London: Taylor & Francis, pp. 925–932.

Khalil, T.M.; Abdel-Moty, E., and Waly, S.M. 1985. "Computerized Signal Processing in the Assessment of Muscular Fatigue." *Computers and Industrial Engineering*, 9(suppl).

Khalil, T.M.; Abdel-Moty, E.; Zaki, A. M.; Dilsen, E.K.; DeVito, C.; Steele-Rosomoff, R.; and Rosomoff, H.L. 1992. "Reducing the Potential for Fall Accidents Among the Elderly Through Physical Restoration." In *Advances in Industrial Ergonomics and Safety IV*. Edited by S. Kumar. London: Taylor & Francis, pp. 1127–1134.

Khalil, T.M.; Abdel-Moty, E.; Zaki, A.M.; Velez, B.; Dilsen, E.K.; Diaz, E.; Steele-Rosomoff, R.; and Rosomoff, H.L. 1992. "Effect of Secondary Gain Issues on Performance and Response to Rehabilitation of Workers Compensation Chronic Low Back Pain Patients." In *Advances in Industrial Ergonomics and Safety IV*. Edited by S. Kumar. London: Taylor & Francis, pp. 1187–1194.

Khalil, T.M.; Asfour, S.S.; Abdel-Moty, E.; Rosomoff, R.S.; and Rosomoff, H.L. 1988. "Quantitative Assessment of Outcome of a Low Back Pain Rehabilitation Program." Abstracts of the International Conference on the Study of the Lumbar Spine, Miami, FL, April 13–15.

Khalil, T.; Asfour, S.; Goldberg, M.; Moty, E.; Fishbain, D.; Santana, R.; Rosomoff, R.; and Rosomoff, H. 1990. "Letter to the Spine," *Spine* 15:4:342–343.

Khalil, T.M.; Asfour, S.S.; Marchette, B.; and Omachonu V. 1987. "Lower Back Injuries in Nursing: A Biomechanical Analysis and Intervention Strategy." In *Trends in Ergonomics/Human Factors IV,* Edited by S.S. Asfour. North-Holland, Amsterdam: Elsevier Science Publishers B.V., pp. 811–821.

Khalil, T.M.; Asfour, S.S.; Martinez, L.M.; Waly, S.M.; Rosomoff, R.S.; and Rosomoff, H.L. 1992. "Stretching in the Rehabilitation of Low Back Pain Patients." *Spine* 17:3:311–317.

Khalil, T.M.; Asfour, S.S.; and Moty, E.A. 1984. "Case Studies in Low Back Pain." Proceedings of the 28th Annual Meeting of the Human Factors Society, pp. 465–468.

———. 1985. "New Horizons for Ergonomics Research in Low Back Pain." In *Trends in Ergonomics/Human Factors II*. Edited by R.E. Eberts and C.G. Eberts. North Holland, Amesterdam: Elsevier Science Publishers B.V., pp. 591–598.

———. 1991. "Clinical Ergonomics: Ergonomic Practice in Health Care Setting." In *Designing for Everyone*. Edited by Y. Queinnec and F. Daniellou. London: Taylor & Francis, pp. 314–316.

Khalil, T.M.; Asfour, S.S.; Moty, E.A.; Goldberg, M.; Steele, R.; and Rosomoff, H.L. 1986. "Acceptable Muscular Effort (AME): An Approach for Assessing Muscular Strength in Low Back Pain Patients." Abstracts of the International Society for the Study of the Lumbar Spine Annual Meeting, Dallas, TX, May 28–June 2.

Khalil, T.M.; Asfour, S.S.; Moty, E.A.; Rosomoff, H.L.; Steele, R., 1983. "The Management of Low Back Pain: A Comprehensive Approach." Proceedings of the Annual Industrial Conference, Louisville, KY, pp. 199–204.

Khalil, T.M.; Asfour, S.S.; Moty, E.A.; Rosomoff, R.S.; and Rosomoff H.L. 1987. "Ergonomics Contribution to Low Back Pain Rehabilitation." *Pain Management*, Sep/Oct:225–230.

Khalil, T.M.; Asfour, S.S.; Moty, E.A.; Steele, R.; and Rosomoff, H.L. 1985. "The Contribution of Ergonomics to Pain Programs." American Pain Society Annual Meeting, Dallas, TX, October 18–20, p. 69.

Khalil, T.M.; Asfour, S.S.; and Waly, S.M. 1988. "Electromyographic Methodologies in Rehabilitation." In *Ergonomics in Rehabilitation.* Edited by A. Mital and W. Karwowski. London: Taylor & Francis, pp. 171–181.

Khalil, T.M.; Asfour, S.S.; Waly, S.M.; Rosomoff, R.S.; and Rosomoff, H.L. 1987. "Effects of Feedback Information on Isometric Training." In *Biomechanics XA.* Edited by B. Johnson. Champaign, Illinois: Human Kinetic Publishers, pp. 491–494.

———. 1987b. "Isometric Exercise and Biofeedback in Strength Training." In *Trends in Ergonomics/Human Factors* IV. Edited by S.S. Asfour. North Holland, Amsterdam: Elsevier Science Publishers, pp. 1095–1101.

———. 1988. "Effectiveness of Aggressive Treatment of Back Rain." In *Trends in Ergonomics/Human Factors* V. Edited by F. Aghazadah. New Holland, Amsterdam: Elsevier Science Publishers, B.V. pp. 997–1983.

Khalil, T.M.; and Ayoub, M.A. 1976. "Work–Rest Scheduling Under Normal and Prolonged Vibration Environments." *Am Indust Hyg Assoc J* March, 233–239.

Khalil, T.; Ayoub, M.; Snook, S.; and Abdel-Moty, E. 1991. "Ergonomic Issues in Low Back Pain: Intervention Strategies." Proceedings of the 35th Annual Meeting of the Human Factors Society, San Francisco, CA, September 2–6, pp. 834–837.

Khalil, T.M.; and Bell, B.H. 1972. "Ergonomics in Dentistry." Proceedings of the 23rd National Meeting of the American Institute of Industrial Engineering Los Angeles, CA pp. 95–100.

———. 1974. "An Ergonomic Investigation in the Design and Use of Hand Instruments." *Quintessence International* March.

Khalil, T.M.; Genaidy, A.M.; Asfour, S.S.; and Vinceguera T. 1985. "Physiologic Limits in Lifting." *Am Indust Hyg Assoc J* 46:4:220–224.

Khalil, T.M.; Goldberg, M.L.; Asfour, S.S.; Moty, E.A.; Steele, R.; and Rosomoff, H.L. 1987. "Acceptable Maximum Effort (AME): A Psychophysical Measure of Strength in Back Pain Patients." *Spine* 12:4:372–376.

Khalil, T.M.; Martinez, A.G.; and Boykin, W.D. 1976. "Electromyographic Models of Mechanical Torque." In *Biomechanics* vol. V. Edited by P.V. Komi. Baltimore: University Park Press.

Khalil, T.M.; and Otero, J.E. 1974. "Processed Muscular Activity During Static and Dynamic Loading." *J Human Ergology* 3:1:75–83.

Khalil, T.M.; and Ramadan, M.Z. 1987. "Biomechanical Evaluation of Lifting Tasks: A Microcomputer-based Model." *Comput Indust Eng* 14:1.

Khalil, T.M.; Truscheit, R.E. 1974. "A Method of Evaluation of the Effectiveness of Dental Operatory Systems." *J Dental Res,* August, pp. 915–924.

Khalil, T.M.; Waly, S.M.; Genaidy, A.M.; and Asfour, S.S. 1987. "Determination of Lifting Abilities: A Comparative Study of Four Techniques." *Am Indust Hyg Assoc J* 48:12:951–956.

Khalil, T.M.; Waly, S.M.; and Zaki, A.M. 1990. "The Effect of Load Expectation on Muscle Recruitment." In *Advances in Industrial Ergonomics and Safety,* vol. II. Edited by B. Das. Taylor & Francis, pp. 159–166.

Khalil, T.M.; and Williams, D.B. 1973. "MTM in the Evaluation of Dental Operatory Design." *J Methods-Time Measur* 18:1.
Kirsch, I. 1986. "Response Expectancy and Phobic Anxiety." *American Pyschol* 41, 1391–1393.
Kopec, J.; Housmanowa-Petrusewicz, I.; Rawski, M.; and Wolynski, M. 1973. "Automated Analysis in Electromyography." In *New Development in Electromyography and Clinical Neurophysiology* vol. 2. Edited by J.E. Desmedt, Karger, Basel: pp. 477–481.
Kores, R.C.; Murphy, W.D.; Rosenthal, T.L.; Elias, D.B.; and North, W.C. 1990. "Predicting Outcome of Chronic Pain Treatment via a Modified Self-efficacy Scale." *Behav Res Ther* 28:2:165–169.
Kornfeld, J. 1982. "Getting Aggressive About Conservative Therapy for Back Pain." *Med World News,* July 5, pp. 68–88.
Kranz, H.; Williams, A.M.; Cassell, J.; Caddy, O.J.; and Silberstein, B. 1983. "Factors Determining the Frequency Content of the Electromyogram." *J Appl Physiol* 55:2:392–399.
Kroemer, K.H.E. 1970. "Human Strength: Terminology, Measurement and Interpretation of Data." *Human Factors* 12:3:297–313.
———. 1983. "An Isoinertial Technique to Assess Individual Lifting Capability." *Human Factors* 25:5:493–506.
Kroemer, K.H.E.; and Robinette, J.C. 1969. "Ergonomics in the Design of Office Furniture." *Indust Med Surg* 38:115.
Lago, P.; and Jones, N. 1977. "Effect of Motor Unit Firing Statistics on EMG Spectra." *Med Biol Eng Comput* 15:648–655.
Lankhorst, G.J.; Stadt, R.J.; and Vogelear, T.W. 1982. "Objectivity and Repeatability of Measurements in Low Back Pain." *Scand J of Rehab Med* 14:21–26.
Laughman, R.K.; and Youdas, J.W. 1983. "Strength Changes in the Normal Quadriceps Femoris Muscle as a Result of Electrical Stimulation." *Phys Ther* 63:4:494–499.
Leavitt, S.S.; Johnson, T.A.; and Bayer, R.D. 1971. "The Process of Recovery Patterns in Industrial Back Injury: 1. Cost and Other Quantitative Measures of Effort." *Ind Med Surg* 40:7–14.
Leavitt, S.; Johnson, T.; and Beyer, R.D. 1982. "Organic Status, Psychological Disturbances and Pain Report: Characteristics in Low Back Pain Patients on Compensation." *Spine* 7:398–402.
LeVeau, B. 1977. *Biomechanics of Human Motion.* Philadelphia: W.B. Sanders.
Lindstrom, L. 1975. "The Myoelectric Power Spectrum: A Model and Its Applications." Proceedings International Workshop on Voluntary Human Motion, Report IWVHM-Proc-75, pp. 69–91.
Locke, T.C. 1983. "Stretching Away from Back Pain Injury." *Occup Health Safety,* July, 52:8–13.
Loser, J.D. 1979. "Low Back Pain: Introduction to Plenary Session." In *Advances in Pain Research and Therapy, vol. III.* Edited by J.J. Bonica. New York: Raven Press, pp. 631–633.
McCaffrey, M. 1980. "Understanding Your Patient's Pain." *Nursing* 80:28-31.

McCormick, E.J.; and Sanders, M.S. 1982. *Human Factors in Engineering and Design,* 5th ed. New York: McGraw-Hill.

McGinnis, G.E.; Seward, M.L.; DeJong, G.; and Osberg, J.S. 1986. "Program Evaluation of Physical Medicine and Rehabilitation Department Using Self-report Barthel." *Arch Phys Med Rehab* 67:123–125.

McMiken, D.F.; Todd-Smith, M.; and Thompson, C. 1983. "Strengthening of Human Quadriceps Muscles by Cutaneous Electrical Stimulation." *Scand J Rehab Med* 15:25–28.

MacNab, I. 1972. "The Mechanisms of Spondylogenic Pain." In *Cervical Pain.* Edited by C. Hirsh and Y. Zotterman. New York: Pergamon Press, p. 89.

Magora, A. 1972. "Investigation of the Relation Between Low Back Pain and Occupation." 3: Physical requirements: Sitting, standing, and weight lifting. *Indus Med Surg* 41:5.

Malec, J.; Cayner, J.J.; Harvey, R.F.; and Timming, G. 1981. "Pain management: Long-term Follow-up of Inpatient Program." *Arch Phys Med Rehab* 62:369–372.

Malone, T.R., ed, 1988. "Ariel Computerized Exercise System." In *Evaluation of Isokinetic Equipment,* vol. 1, no. 1. Baltimore: Williams & Wilkins.

Marras, W; King, A; and Joynt, R. 1984. "Measurement of Loads on the Lumbar Spine Under Isometric and Isokinetic Conditions." *Spine* 9:176–187.

Marras, W.S.; Rangarjulu, S.L.; and Lavender, S., 1987. "Trunk Loading and Expectation." *Ergonomics* 30:551–556.

Massey, B.H.; Nelson, R.C.; Sharkey, B.C.; and Comden, T. 1965. "Effects of High Frequency Electrical Stimulation on the Size and Strength of Skeletal Muscle." *J Sports Med Phys Fitness* 5:136–144.

Matheson, L.N.; Ogden, L.D.; Violette, K; Schultz, K. 1985. "Work Hardening: Occupational Therapy in Industrial Rehabilitation." *Am J Occup Ther* 39:5:314–319.

Mayer, T.G. 1985. "Using the Physical Measurements to Assess Low Back Pain." *J Musculoskel Med* 2:44–59.

Mayer, T.G.; and Gatchel, R.J. 1988. "Functional Restoration for Spinal Disorders: The Sports Medicine Approach." Philadelphia: Lea & Febiger.

Mayer, T.G.; Gatchel, R.J.; Kishino, N; Keeley, J.; Capra, P.; Mayer, H.; Barnett, and Moorey, V. 1985. "Objective Assessment of Spine Function Following Industrial Injury (A Prospective Study with Comparison Group and one-year follow-up.) *Spine* 10:6:482–493.

Mayer, T.G.; Gatchel, R.J.; Kishino, N.; Keeley, J.; Mayer, H.; Capra, P.; and Mooney, V. 1986. A Prospective Short-term Study of Chronic Low Back Pain Patients Utilizing Novel Objective Functional Measurement." *Pain* 25:1:53–68.

Mayer, T.G.; Smith, S.S.; Keeley, J., Mooney, V. 1985. "Quantification of Lumbar Function. Part 2: Saggital Plane Trunk Strength in Chronic Low Back Pain Patients." *Spine* 10:8:765–772.

Mayer, T.G.; Tencer, A.F.; Kristoferson, S.; and Mooney, V. 1984. "Use of Noninvasive Technique for Quantification of Spinal Ranges of Motion in Normal Subjects and Chronic Low Back Dysfunction Patients." *Spine* 9:588–595.

Mehler, W.R. 1966. "Some Observations on Secondary Ascending Afferent Systems in the Central Nervous System." In *Pain* (Henry Ford Hospital International

Symposium). Edited by R.S. Knight, P.R. Dumke. Boston: Little Brown & Co., pp. 11–32.

Mellin, G, 1989. "Chronic Low Back Pain Med 54–63 Years of Age. Correlation of Physical Measurements With the Degree of Trouble and Progress After Treatment." *Spine* 11:5:421–426.

Melton, B. 1983. "Back Injury Prevention Means Education." *Occup Health Safety* 52:20–23.

Merletti, R.; Andina, A.; Galante, M.; and Furlan, I. 1979. "Clinical Experience of Electronic Peroneal Stimulators in 50 Hemiparetic Patients." *Scand J Rehab Med* 11:111–119.

Merskey, H. 1986. "Classification of Chronic Pain: Descriptions of Chronic Pain Syndromes and Definitions of Pain Terms." *Pain* 3(suppl):226.

Mixter, W.J.; and Barr, J.S. 1934. "Rupture of the Intervertebral Disc with Involvement of the Spinal Canal." *N Eng J Med* 211:210–215.

Morris, J.M.; Lucas, D.B.; and Bresler, B. 1961. "Role of the Trunk in Stability of the Spine." *J Bone Joint Surg* 43A:327–351.

Moty, E.A.; and, Khalil, T.M. 1984. "The Application of Information Theory in EMG Processing." Proceedings of the 37th Annual Conference on Engineering in Medicine and Biology, Los Angeles, CA, p. 73.

———. 1987. "Computerized Signal Processing Techniques for the Quantification of Muscular Activity." *Comput Indust Eng* 12:3:193–203.

Nachemson, A.L. 1971. "Low Back Pain: Its Etiology and Treatment." *Clin Med* pp. 78:18–23.

———. 1976. "The Lumbar Spine: An Orthopedic Challenge." *Spine* 1:59–71.

Nachemson, A. 1981. "Toward a Better Understanding of Low Back Injury." Liberty Mutual Back Pain Symposium, Boston, MA, pp. 4–13.

Nachemson, A.L.; and Elfstrom, E. 1970. "Intravital Dynamic Pressure Measurements in Lumbar Discs. A Study of Common Movements, Maneuvers, and Exercises." *Scand J Rehab Med* 2 (suppl 1):1–40.

Nachemson, A.L.; and Lindh, M. 1969. "Measurement of Abdominal and Back Muscle Strength with and without Low Back Pain." *Scand J Rehab Med* 1:60–69.

National Center for Health Statistics. 1985. "Low Back Pain: What Is the Best Conservative Management." *Data Centrum* 2:15–29.

National Institute for Occupational Safety and Health (NIOSH). 1981. "A Work Practice Guide for Manual Lifting." Technical report #81-122, U.S. Dept. of Health and Human Services, Cincinnati, OH.

Nemeth, P.M. 1982. "Electrical Stimulation of Denervated Muscle Prevents Decreases in Oxidative Enzymes." *Muscle-Nerve* 5:2:134–139.

Newman, R.I.; Seres, J.L.; Yospe, L.P.; and Garlington, B. 1978. "Multidisciplinary Treatment of Chronic Pain: Long-term Follow-up of Low Back Patients." *Pain* 4:283–292.

Nordby, E.J. 1981. "Epidemiology and Diagnosis of Low Back Injury." Occup Health & Safety, January, pp. 38–41.

Novak, J. 1981. "The Back Loser." Liberty Mutual Back Pain Symposium, Boston, MA, pp. 52–57.

Ng, L.K.Y., ed. 1981. "New Approaches to Treatment of Chronic Pain: A Review of

Multidisciplinary Pain Clinics and Pain Centers." Washington, DC, U.S. Government Printing Office. Monograph # 36.

Oborne, D.J. 1987. *Ergonomics at Work,* 2nd ed. Bath, England: Bath Press.

Oort, G.V.; Frederick, M.; Pinto, D.; and Ragone, D. 1990. "Back Injuries Require Integration of Aggressive and Passive Treatment." Occup Health & Safety, January, pp. 22–24.

Osterweis, A; Kleinman, A.; and Mechan, D. (eds). 1987. "Pain and Disability." In *Clinical, Behavioral and Public Policy Perspectives.* Institute of Medicine, Committee on Pain Disability and Chronic Illness Behavior. Washington, DC: National Academy Press.

Owens, J.; and Malone, T. 1983. "Treatment Parameters of High Frequency Electrical Stimulation as Established on the Electro-Stim 180." *J Orthop Sports Phys Ther* 4:3:162–168.

Park, K.S.; and Chaffin, D.B. 1974. "A Biomechanical Evaluation of Two Methods of Manual Load Lifting." *Am Inst. Indus Eng Transactions Trans* 6:2:105–113.

Petherick, M.; Rheault, W.; Kimble, S.; Lechner, C.; and Senear, V. 1988. "Concurrent Validity and Intertester Reliability of Universal and Fluid Based Goniometers for Active Elbow Range of Motion." *Phys Ther* 68:966–969.

Pheasant, H. 1977. "Backache—Its Nature, Incidence and Cost." *West J Med* 126:330–332.

Pisciotta, J.C. 1987. Unpublished report comparing the Orthoranger II electrogoniometer and the standard goniometer. Ohio State University, Gait Analysis Laboratory.

Pope, M.H.; Frymoyer, J.W.; and Andersson, G. 1984. *Occupational Low Back Pain.* New York: Praeger Publishers.

Pope, M.H.; Wilder, D.G.; Stokes, I.A.F.; and Frymore, J.W. 1979. "Biomechanical Testing as an Aid to Decision Making in Low Back Pain Patients." *Spine* 4:2:135–140.

Pytel, J.L.; and Kamon, E. 1981. "Dynamic Strength as a Predictor of Maximal and Acceptable Lifting." *Ergonomics* 24:9:663–672.

Quebec Study. 1987. "Scientific Approach to the Assessment and Management of Activity-related Spinal Disorders: A Monograph for Clinicians." (Report of Quebec Task Force on Spinal Disorders.) *Spine* 12:75.

Rashwan, A; Khalil, T.M.; and Moty, E.A. 1984. "Computerized Signal Analysis Techniques in Electromography." *Egypt J Biomed Eng* 3:1–2:1–20

Rintala, D.H.; and Willems, E.P. 1991. "Telephone versus Face-to-Face Mode for Collecting Self-reports of Sequences of Behavior." *Arch Phys Med Rehab* 72:477–481.

Rodgers, S.H. 1984. *Working with Backache.* Fairport, New York: Perinton Press.

———.1988. "Job Evaluation in Worker's Fitness Determination." *Occup Med* 3:2:219–239.

Roland, M.; and Morris, R. 1983. "Development of Reliable and Sensitive Measure of Disability in Low Back Pain." *Spine* 8:2:663–672.

Romero, J.A.; Sanford, T.L.; Schroeder, R.V.; and Fahey. 1982. "The Effects of Electrical Stimulation of Normal Quadriceps on Strength and Girth." *Med Sci Sports Exer* 14:3:194–197.

Rose, A.; and Willison, R. 1967. "Quantifying Electromyography Using Automated Analysis: Studies in Healthy Subjects and Patients with Primary Muscle Disease." *J Neurol Neurosurg Psychiatr* 30:403–410.

Rosomoff, H.L. 1985a. "Do Herniated Disks Produce Pain?" *Clin J Pain* 1:91–93.

———. 1985b. "Non-operative treatment of the Failed Back Syndrome Presenting with Chronic Pain." In *Current Therapy in Neurosurgery.* Edited by D. Long, Toronto: B.C. Decker, pp. 200–202

———. 1987. "Comprehensive Pain Center Approach to the Treatment of Low Back Pain." In *Low back pain.* Report of a workshop, Rehabilitation Research and Training Center, Department Orthopedic Rehababilation, University of Virginia, pp. 78–85.

Rosomoff, H.L.; Clasen, R.A.; Hartstock, R, et al., 1965. "Brain Reaction to Experimental Injury After Hypothermia." *Arch Neurol* 13:337–345.

Rosomoff, H; Fishbain, D.; Cutler, B.; Abdel-Moty, E.; and Steele-Rosomoff, R. 1991. "Pain Center Treatment Outcome for the 'Failed Back Syndrome.' " Abstracts of the American Pain Society Meeting, November 7–10, New Orleans, LA, p. 117.

Rosomoff, H.L.; Fishbain, D.A.; Goldberg, M.; Santana, R.; and Rosomoff-Steele, R. 1989. "Physical Findings in Patients with Chronic Intractable Benign Pain of the Neck and/or Back." *Pain* 37(3):279–287.

Rosomoff, H.L.; Fishbain, O.A.; Goldberg, M.L.; and Steele-Rosomoff, R. 1990. "Myofascial Findings in Patients with Chronic Intractable Benign Pain of the Back and Neck." *Pain Management*, March/April, pp 114–118.

Rosomoff, H.L.; Green, C.; Silbert, M.; and Steele, R. 1981. "Pain and Low Back Rehabilitation Program at the University of Miami School of Medicine." In *New Approaches to Treatment of Chronic Pain: A Review of Multidisciplinary Pain Clinics and Pain Centers.* Edited by K.Y. Lorenzo. NIDA Research Monograph 36, Department of HHS, pp. 92–111.

Rosomoff, H.L.; Rosomoff, R.S.; 1987. "Non-surgical Aggressive Treatment of Lumbar Spinal Stenosis." In *Spine: State of the Art Reviews,* Vol. 1, No. 3. Philadelphia: Hanley and Belfus, pp. 383–400.

———. 1991. "Comprehensive Multidisciplinary Pain Center Approach to the Treatment of Low Back Pain." In *Neurosurgery Clinics of North America*, vol. 2, no. 4, pp. 877–890.

Rosomoff, H.L.; Steele-Rosomoff, R. 1988. "Pain Management Programs for Low Back Disorders." *Miami Med*, March, 25–26.

Rosomoff, R.S. 1991. "The Pain Patient." In *Spine: State of the Art Reviews,* vol. 5, no. 3, pp. 417–427.

Rothstein, J.M.; Miller, P.J.; and Roettger, R.F. 1983. "Goniometric Reliability in a Clinical Setting." *Phys Ther* 63:1611–1615.

Rowe, M.L. 1969. "Low Back Pain in Industry." *J Occup Med* 11:4:161–169.

———. 1983. *Backache at Work.* Fairport, New York: Perinton Press.

Roy, S.H.; DeLuca, C.J.; Casavant, D.A. 1989. Lumbar Muscle Function and Chronic Lower Back Pain. *Spine* 14:9:992–1001.

Roy, S.H.; DeLuca, C.J.; and Gilmore, L.D. 1986. "Computer-aided Back Analysis System." Proceedings of the 8th Annual Conference of IEEE-EMBS, Dallas–Fort Worth, TX, November 8.

Rutkow, I.M. 1986. "Orthopaedic Operations in the United States, 1979 through 1983." *J Bone Joint Surg* 68A:716–719.

Sadoyama, T.; Masuda, T.; and Miyano, H. 1983. "Relationship Between Muscle Fiber Conduction Velocity and Frequency Parameters of Surface EMG During Sustained Contractions." *Eur J Appl Physiol* 51:247–256.

Sanders, S.H. 1980. "Toward Instrument System for the Automatic Measurement of 'uptime' in Chronic Pain Patients." *Pain* 9:103–109.

Sato, H. 1982. "Functional Characteristic of Human Skeletal Muscle Revealed by Spectral Analysis of Surface EMG." *Electromyogr Clin Neurophysiol* 22:459–516.

Schaepe, J.L. 1982. "Low Back Pain: An Occupational Perspective." In *Chronic Low Back Pain*. Edited by M. Stanton-Hicks and R. Boas. New York: Raven Press, pp.1–13.

Schultz, A.B.; Andersson, G.B.J.; Haderspeek, K.; Nachemson, A. 1982. "Loads on the Lumbar Spine." *J Bone Joint Surg* 64A:713–720.

Schultz, A.; and Haderspeck, K. 1981. "Correction of Scoliosis by Muscle Stimulation: Biomechanical Analysis." *Spine* 6:5:468–476.

Selkowitz, D.W. 1985. "Improvement in Isometric Strength of the Quadriceps Femoris Muscle After Training with Electrical Stimulation." *Phys Ther,* 65:2:186–196.

Simons, D.G.; and Travell, J.G. 1983. "Myofascial Origins of Low Back Pain," Parts I & II. *Postgrad Med* 73:66–108.

Smidt, G.; Herring, T.; Amundsen, L.; Rogers, M.; Russell, A.; and Lehmann, T. 1983. "Assessment of Abdominal and Back Extension Functions: A Quantitative Approach." *Spine* 8:2:211–219.

Smyth, M.J.; and Wright, V. 1985. "Sciatica and the Intervertebral Disc." An experimental study. *J Bone Joint Surg* 40A:1401–1418.

Snook, S.H.; 1978. The Design of Manual Handling Tasks. *Ergonomics* 21:12:963–985.

Snook, S.H. 1983. Low Back Pain in Industry. Proc. Workshop Idiopathic Low Back Pain. White & Gordon, C.V. Mosby, pp. 23–38.

———. 1982. "Low Back Pain in Industry." In *Symposium on Idiopathic Low Back Pain*. Edited by A.A. White III and S.L. Gordon. St Louis: C.V. Mosby, pp.23–37.

Snook, S.H.; Campanelli, R.; and Hart, J. 1978. "A Study of Three Preventive Approaches to Low Back Injury." *J of Occup Med* 20:478–481.

Snook, S.H.; and Ciriello, V.M. 1974. Maximum Weights and Work Loads Acceptable to Female Workers. *J Occup Med* 16:527–534.

Snook, S.H., and Irvine, C.H. 1967. "Maximum Acceptable Weight of Lift." *Am Indust Hyg Assoc J,* 9:322–329.

Snook, S.H.; Irvine, C.H.; and Bass S.F. 1970. "Maximum Weights and Workloads Acceptable to Male Industrial Workers." *Am Indust Hyg Assoc J,* 71:579–586.

Snook, S.H.; Jensen, R.C. 1984. "Cost of Occupational Low Back Pain." In *Occupational Low Back Pain*. Edited by M.H. Pope, J.W. Frymoyer and G. Anderson. New York: Praeger Publishers, pp. 115–121.

Social Security Administration, 1986. Report of the Commission on Evaluation of Pain. Department of Health and Human Resources, Washington, DC.

Spektor, S. 1990. "Chronic Pain and Pain Related Disabilities." *J Disab* 1:2:98–102.

Spiegel, Z.S., Hirshfield, M.S., and Spiegel, T.M. 1985. "Evaluating Self-care Activities: Comparison of a Self-reported Questionnaire with an Occupational Therapist Interview." *British J Rheumatol* 24:357–361.

Spitzer, W.O.; LeBlanc, F.E.; Dupuis, M, 1987. "Scientific Approach to the Assessment and Management of Activity Related Spinal Disorders: A Monograph for Clinicians." (Report of the Quebec Task Force on Spinal Disorders.) *Spine* 12(suppl 1):51–59.

Standish, W.D.; and Valiant, G. 1981. "The Effects of Immobilization and of Electrical Stimulation on Muscle Glycogen and Myofibrillar ATP-ase." Presented at the American Academy of Orthopedic Surgeons, Las Vegas. NV.

Stanton-Hicks, M.; and Boas R. 1982. *Chronic Low Back Pain.* New York: Raven Press.

Steele, R. 1984. "Is the Pain Team Cost Effective?" *Pain* 2(suppl):438.

Steele-Rosomoff, R.; Fishbain, D.; Goldberg, M.; Culter, B.; Abdel-Moty, E.; Steele-Rosomoff, R.; and Rosomoff, H. 1991. "Pain Patients Who Lie in Their Psychiatric Examination About Current Drug/Alcohol Use." Abstracts of the American Pain Society Meeting, November 7–10, New Orleans, LA, p. 130.

Steinberg, G.G. 1982. "Epidemiology of Low Back Pain." In *Chronic Low Back Pain* Edited by M. Stanton-Hicks and R. Boas New York: Raven Press, pp. 1–14.

Stulen, F.B.; and DeLuca, C.J. 1981. "Frequency Parameters of the Myoelectric Signal as a Measure of Muscle Conduction Velocity." *IEEE Trans Biomed Eng* BME-28:515–523.

Susser, M. 1990. "Disease, Illness, Sickness, Impairment, Disability and Handicap." *Psychol Med* 20:471–473.

Suzuki, N.; and Endo, S. 1983. "A Quantitative Study of Trunk Muscle Strength and Fatigability in Low Back Pain Syndrome." *Spine* 8:211–216.

Svensson, H.; and Andersson, G. 1983. "Low Back Pain in 40-to 47-Year Old-Men: Work History and Environment Factors." *Spine* 8:272–276.

Takebe, K.; Kukulka, C.; and Marayan, M.G. 1975. "Peroneal Nerve Stimulation in Rehabilitation of Hemiplegic Patients." *Arch Phys Med* 56:237–240.

Task Force on Guidelines for Desirable Characteristics for Pain Treatment Facilities Standards for Physicians Fellowship in Pain Management. 1990. International Association for the Study of Pain, Seattle, WA.

Thompson, M.C.; Shingleton, L.G.; and Kegerries, S.T. 1989. "Comparison of Values Generated During Testing of the Knee the Cybex II Plus and Biodex Model B-2000 Isokinetic Dynamometer." *JOSPT.* 11:3:108–115.

Tichaur, E.R. 1979. *The Biomechanical Basis of Ergonomics.* New York: John Wiley & Sons.

Travell, J.; and Rinzler, S.H. 1952. "The Myofascial Genesis of Pain." *Post Grad Med* 11:425–434.

Travell, J.G.; and Simons, D.G. 1983. *Myofascial Pain and Dysfunction: The Trigger Point Manual.* Baltimore: Williams & Wilkins.

Trief, P.M. 1983. "Chronic Back Pain: A Tripatite Model of Outcome." *Arch Phys Med Rehab* 64:53–56.

Troup, J.D.G. 1965. "The relation of Lumbar Spine Disorder to Heavy Manual Work and Lifting." *Lancet* 1:857–861.

———. 1978. "Driver's Back Pain and Its Prevention: A Review of the Postural,

Vibratory and Muscular Factors Together with the Problem of Transmitted Road Shocks." *Appl Ergonomics* 78:207–214.

Turk, R.; and Kralj, A. 1980. "The Alteration of Paraplegic Patients Muscle Properties due to Electrical Stimulation Exercising." *Paraplegia* 18:6:386–391.

USDOL (U.S. Department of Labor), Employment and Training Administration. 1977. *Dictionary of Occupational Titles*, 4th ed, Washington, DC: U.S. Government Printing Office.

———. 1981. *Selected Characteristics of Occupations Defined in the DOT.* Washington, DC: U.S. Government Printing Office.

———. 1982a. *Dictionary of Occupational Titles*, 4th ed, Washington, DC: U.S. Government Printing Office.

———. 1982b. *A Guide to Job Analysis.* Washington, DC: U.S. Government Printing Office.

———. 1986. *Dictionary of Occupational Titles*, 4th ed, Washington, DC: U.S. Government Printing Office.

U.S. News and World Report, 1987. "Taking the Pain Out of Pain." Horizons, June 29, pp. 50–57.

Van Overeem Hanson, G. 1979. "Controlled Functional Electrical Stimulation of the Paretic Hand." *Scand J Rehab Med* 11:4:189–193.

Vane, J.R. 1983. "Pain of Inflammation: An Introduction." In *Advances in Pain Research and Therapy.* Edited by J.J. Bonica. New York: Raven Press, p. 597.

Vital and Health Statistics. 1974. Limitations of Activity due to Chronic Conditions, series 10, no. 111. Department of Health, Education, and Welfare, Washington, DC.

———. 1977. Utilization of Short-stay Hospitals. Annual Summary of the United States, Series 13, no 41. U.S. Department of Health, Education and Welfare, Washington, DC.

Waddell, G. 1987. "A New Clinical Model for the Treatment of Low-back Pain." *Spine* 12:532–644.

Waddell, G.; Kummel, E.G.; Lotto, W.N.; 1979. "Failed Lumbar Disc Surgery and Repeat Surgery Following Industrial Injuries." *J Bone Joint Surg* 61A:201–207.

Waddell, G.; and Main, C.J. 1984. "Assessment of Severity in Low Back Pain." *Spine* 9:2:204–208.

———. 1980. "The Role of Substantia Gelatinosa as a Gate Control." In *Pain.* Edited by J.J. Bonica. New York: Raven Press, p. 205.

Wall PD, 1974. "Physiological Mechanism Involved in the Production and Relief of Pain." In *Recent Advances on Pain: Pathophysiology and Clinical Aspects.* Edited by J.J. Bonica, P. Procacci, and C. Pagni. Springfield, Illinois: Charles C Thomas, p. 36.

Weisel, S.W.; Feffer, H.L.; Rothman, R.H. 1985a. "Industrial Low Back Pain. A Prospective Evaluation of a Standardized Diagnostic and Treatment Protocol." *Spine*, 9:199–203.

———. 1985b. *Industrial Low Back Pain.* Charlottesville, Virginia: Michie Law Publishers.

Woodson, W.E. 1981. *Human Factors Design Handbook.* New York: McGraw-Hill.

Zaki, A.M.; Goldberg, M.L.; Khalil, T.M. Jarett, J.; Rodriguez, E.; Linial, A.;

Rosomoff, R.; and Rosomoff, H. 1990. "Comparison Between the One and Two Inclinometer Techniques for Measuring Range of Motion." In *Advances in Industrial Ergonomics and Safety* vol. II, Edited by B. Das. New York: Taylor & Francis, pp. 135–142.

Zaki, A.M.; Khalil, T.M.; Abdel-Moty, E.; Steele-Rosomoff, R.; and Rosomoff, H.L. 1992. "Profile of Chronic Pain Patients and Their Rehabilitation Outcome." In *Advances in Industrial Ergonomics and Safety,* vol. IV. Edited by S. Kumar, London: Taylor & Francis, pp. 1179–1186.

Appendix A
Conversion Factors

ANGLES

1 degree	$= 1.745 \times 10^{-2}$ radians
1 radian	$= 57.29$ degrees

ANGULAR VELOCITY

1 degree per second	$= 1.745 \times 10^{-2}$ radians/sec
	$= 0.1667$ revolutions per minute

AREA

1 square foot	$= 144$ square inches
	$= 2.296 \times 10^{-5}$ acres
	$= 0.092903$ square meters
1 square meter	$= 10.76$ square feet
	$= 0.3861 \times 10^{-8}$ square miles
1 square yard	$= 9$ square feet
	$= 0.8361$ square meters
1 square mile	$= 640$ acres
1 acre	$= 4840$ square yards
	$= 43560$ square feet
1 square centimeter	$= 1.076 \times 10^{-3}$ square feet
	$= 0.155$ square inches
1 square inch	$= 645.16$ square millimeter

ENERGY AND WORK

1 erg	$= 1.0$ dyne-centimeters
	$= 7.376 \times 10^{-8}$ foot-pounds
	$= 3.725 \times 10^{-14}$ horsepower-hours

	$= 1.0 \times 10^{-7}$ joules
	$= 2.773 \times 10^{-4}$ kilowatt hours
1 foot pound	$= 1.355818$ joules
	$= 0.1383$ kilogram-meters
1 kilogram-meter	$= 7.23$ foot-pounds
1 kilocalorie	$= 4.1868$ kilojoules
	$= 3086$ foot-pound
	$= 426.4$ kilogram-meter
1 kilojoules	$= 1000$ joules
	$= 0.23892$ kilocalorie
1 liter oxygen consumed	$= 5.05$ kilocalorie
	$= 15.575$ foot-pounds
	$= 2153$ kilogram-meter
	$= 21.237$ kilojoules
1 MET	$= 3.5$ ml oxygen/Kg-min
	$= 0.0175$ kilocalorie/kilogram

FORCE

1 Newton	$= 1 \text{ Kg} \times \text{m} \times \sec^{-2}$
	$= 1 \times 10^{5}$ dynes
	$= 0.1019$ kilopound
	$= 0.2248$ pound force
1 kilogram force	$= 9.80665$ newton
1 dyne	$= 1.020 \times 10^{-3}$ grams
	$= 1.020 \times 10^{-6}$ kilograms
	$= 2.248 \times 10^{-6}$ pounds
1 pound force	$= 4.448222$ newton

LENGTH

1 inch	$= 25.4$ millimeter
	$= 2.54$ centimeter
	$= 1.578 \times 10^{-5}$ miles
	$= 2.778 \times 10^{-2}$ yards
1 centimeter	$= 3.281 \times 10^{-2}$ feet
	$= 0.3937$ inches
	$= 1 \times 10^{-5}$ kilometers
	$= 6.214 \times 10^{-6}$ miles
	$= 1.094 \times 10^{-2}$ yards
1 foot	$= 30.48$ centimeter
	$= 3.948 \times 10^{-4}$ kilometers
	$= 12$ inches
	$= 0.3048$ meters
1 yard	$= 3$ feet
	$= 0.9144$ meters

1 meter	= 3.281 feet
	= 39.37 inches
	= 1.094 yards
1 mile	= 1609.334 meters
	= 5280 feet
	= 1760 yards
	= 1.61 kilometers
1 kilometer	= 0.62 mile

MASS

1 ounce	= 28.3495 grams
1 pound	= 0.453592 kilograms
1 slug	= 14.5939 kilograms

MOMENT OF INERTIA

1 pound foot squared	= 0.042140 kilogram meters squared

PRESSURE

1 poundal per square foot	= 1.488164 Pa
1 pound-force per square foot	= 47.88026 Pa
1 mm mercury	= 133.322387 Pa

POWER

1 horsepower (metric)	= 745.499 watts
	= 33000 foot-pounds/min
	= 4564 kilogram-meter/min
1 watt	= 44.27 foot-pounds/min
	= 6.118 kilogram-meter/min
	= 0.0013 horsepower
1 foot-pound/minute	= 0.1383 kilogram-meter/min
	= 0.0266 watts
	= 3.03×10^{-5} horsepower

TEMPERATURE

0°C	= 32 °F
100 °C	= 212 °F
°C	= (°F-32) × (5/9)
°F	= [(9/5)(°C)] + 32

TIME

1 day	= 8.64×10^4 seconds
	= 1.44×10^3 minutes

TORQUE

1 Nm	= 0.73756 lb.ft
1 cm. dyne	= 1.020×10^{-3} centimeter-grams
	= 1.020×10^{-8} meter-kilograms
	= 7.375×10^{-8} pound-feet
1 pound foot	= 1.356×10^{7} centimeter-grams

VELOCITY

1 inch per second	= 25.4 meter/sec
1 foot per second	= 0.3048 meter/sec
	= 18.3 meter/min
	= 1.1 kilometer/hour
	= 0.68 mile/hour
1 mile per hour	= 0.45 meter/sec
	= 1.47 foot/sec
	= 26.8 meter/min
	= 1.61 kilometer/hour
1 kilometer per hour	= 16.7 meter/min
	= 0.28 meter/sec
	= 0.62 mile/hour
1 knot	= 6.080×10^{3} feet/hour
	= 1.8532 kilometers/hour

VOLUME

1 cubic centimeter	= 3.531×10^{-5} cubic feet
	= 6.102×10^{-2} cubic inches
	= 1.308×10^{-6} cubic yards
	= 2.642×10^{-4} gallons
	= 1.057×10^{-3} quarts
	= 1×10^{-3} liters
1 cubic inch	= 16.387064 cubic centimeters
1 cubic foot	= 2.832×10^{4} cubic centimeter
	= 1.728×10^{3} cubic inches
	= 3.704×10^{-2} cubic yards
	= 7.481 gallons
	= 29.92 quarts
	= 28.32 liters
1 cubic yard	= 27 cubic feet
	= 0.764555 cubic meters

WEIGHT

1 kilogram	= 2.2046 pounds
	= 9.80665×10^{5} dynes

	= 35.274 ounces
	= 1000 grams
1 quart	= 2 pints
1 gallon	= 4 quarts
	= 3.785 liters
1 ounce	= 16 drams
	= 0.0625 pounds
	= 28.35 grams
1 ounces (fluid)	= 2.96 × 10^{-2} liters
1 pint	= 0.125 gallons
	= 0.4732 liters
1 pound	= 16 ounces
	= 4.448 × 10^5 dynes
	= 0.454 kilograms
	= 454 grams
1 ton	= 2000 pounds
1 slug	= 14.59 kilograms
	= 32.17 pounds
1 gram	= 0.035 ounces
	= 0.0022 pound

Appendix B
Constants and Multipliers

Acceleration of gravity (g)   = 32.17 ft/sec^2
Velocity of sound   = 33136 cm/sec
Velocity of light (c)   = 299790200000 cm/sec
PI   = 3.14159265

gega	10^9	mega	10^6	kilo	10^3
centi	10^{-2}	milli	10^{-3}	micro	10^{-6}
nano	10^{-9}				

Appendix C

Biomechanical Definitions and Formulas

Physical Quantity	Description
Biomechanics	The application of laws of Newtonian mechanics to the human body.
Center of Gravity	The single point of the body about which every particle of its mass is equally distributed. For humans, the CG is slightly anterior to the S2 vertebrae.
Concentric Contraction	Shortening of the muscle to aid movement.
Dynamics	The mechanics of the body as it accelerates or decelerates.
Eccentric Contraction	Lengthening of the muscle to slow movement.
Forces Affecting Motion	Gravity, muscle tension, external resistance, and friction.
Frequency	The number of repetitions of a periodic event that occur in a given time interval. ($f = 1/T = w/2PI$ where T is the time to complete one cycle of the event, w is the angular frequency (time rate of change of orientation of a line segment in radians per second), and $PI = 3.141$.
Force	The mechanical action or effect of one body on another, which causes the bodies to accelerate relative to an inertial reference frame. One newton is

Biomechanical Definitions and Formulas 215

that force that when applied to a one kilogram mass causes it to accelerate at one meter per second in the direction of force application and relative to the inertial reference frame:
$1 N = 1 Kg \cdot m \cdot s^{-2}$

Isometric Contraction — The muscle contracts and produces force without changing the angle of the joint.

Isotonic Contraction — A condition where the muscle contracts while maintaining constant effort.

Isokinetic Contraction — Contraction occurring at a constant rate.

Kinematics — The description of the positions and motions of the body in space.

Kinesiology — The study of motion.

Kinetic Energy (T) — Energy of motion. $T = m \cdot v^2/2$ where m=mass and v=velocity. for a rigid body: $T = m \cdot v^2/2 + I \cdot w^2/2$ where I = mass moment of inertia = $Kg \cdot m^2$.

Kinetics — The description of the forces that produce, arrest, or modify motion of the body.

Statics — The mechanics of the body at rest or in uniform motion.

Mechanical Energy (E) — The capacity to do work.
E = potential energy + kinetic energy

Newton's First Law — Every body persists in its state of rest or of uniform motion in a straight line unless it is compelled to change that state by forces impressed on it.

Newton's Second Law — The acceleration of a body is proportional to the magnitude of the resultant forces on it and inversely proportional to the mass of the body.

Potential Energy (V) — Energy due to position. The gravitational potential energy of a mass (m) raised a distance (h) above some reference level: $V = m \times g \times h$, where g is the acceleration due to gravity.

Torque — The product of a force times the perpendicular distance from its line of action to the axis of motion: $T = F \times d$. If the torque produces a clockwise motion, it is positive. If the torques produces a counterclockwise motion,

	it is negative. If the body is in equilibrium, the sum of all torques is zero.
Power (P)	The rate at which work is done or energy is expended. $P = \text{Force} \times \text{Velocity}$ of the point of application of force. Power generated by a moment = moment $\times$ angular velocity of the rigid body.
Power of Contraction	The rate at which muscle work is done: Power = Force or Load $\times$ Speed = Force or Load $\times$ (Distance/Time)
Weight (G)	The force of gravitational attraction acting on a body: $G = m \cdot g$ where m is the mass and g is the acceleration due to gravity.
Work (W)	Work is done when a force acts through a displacement in the direction of the force: $W = \text{force} \times \text{displacement}$.

Appendix D
Body Weight Segments

Percentage Weights of Body Segments

Head	6.9%
Head and Neck	7.9%
Head, Neck, and Trunk	59%
Arm	2.7%
Forearm	1.6%
Hand	0.6%
Upper Limb	4.9%
Forearm & Hand	2.2%
Thigh	9.7%
Leg	4.5%
Foot	1.4%
Lower Limb	15.6%
Leg and Foot	6%

Appendix E
Key To Job Demands

Time Demand Classification

In an eight-hour work day, with (two) 15-minute breaks and a 30-minute meal break, the terms used to describe the frequency of performing a given task are:

Occasional	1–33% of the total time
Frequent	34–66% of the total time
Continuous	67–100% of the total time
Never	0% of the total time

Frequency of Lifting and Carrying

Occasional	1 lift every 30 min
Frequent	1 lift every 2 min
Continuous	1 lift every 15 sec

Lifting Demands for Various Job Categories

	Occasional	Frequent	Continuous
Sedentary	10 or less	Negligible	Negligible
Light	20	10	Negligible
Medium	50	25	10
Heavy	100	50	20
Very Heavy	100+	50+	20+

Index

A

Abilities, 6
Acceptable maximum effort, 113, 144, 145
Achievement scale, 7
Activities of daily living, 136
Acute pain, 31
Adjustability, 64
Anthropometry, 106
    Average person, 68
    Dynamic, 107
    Measures, 106, 108
    Static, 107
Anxiety, 32
Appendicular skeleton, 15
Assessment, 103, 142, 178
Axial skeleton, 14

B

Back support, 60, 85
Balance, 120
Bed rest, 45
Belts, 85
Biofeedback, 147
Biomechanical
    Imbalance, 25
    Models, 88, 90, 167
    Stresses, 87
Body mechanics, 94, 165
Body segments, 212

C

Capacities, 6, 51
Cardiopulmonary, 126
Carrying, 138
Casters, 61
Central nervous system, 109
Chairs, 60
    Back angle, 60
    Back rest, 60
    Casters, 61
    Design guidelines, 60
    Elbow rest, 61
    Height, 60
    Material, 61
    Seat, 60
    Width, 60
Chronic pain, 31
Clinical ergonomics, 48
Compression fractures, 24
Computer-aided design, 66
Concentric, 129
Constants, 213

Contractures, 74
Conversion factors, 208
Cushions, 84

D

Deconditioning, 144
Depression, 28, 32
Design, 5
   Guidelines, 60, 64
   Principles, 60, 64
Disability, 32, 34, 106
Drugs, 33
Dynamic, 93, 128

E

Eccentric, 129
Elbow support, 61
Electromyography, 131, 174
   and Expectation, 180
   Applications, 135, 164
   Needle and Surface, 131
   Processing techniques, 131
Endurance, 130
Energy, 82, 123
Environment, 4, 55
Ergonomics, 1
   Basis, 3
   Concepts, 2
   Role, 7
   Scope, 2
   Contributions 36, 48
   Interventions, 53, 55, 73, 87, 94, 101, 147, 152, 154
   Design, 55, 68, 71
   Job analysis, 55, 154, 162
Evaluation, 103, 139
   Final, 173
   Initial, 173
   Occupational therapy, 39
   Physical therapy, 38
   Physician's, 38
   Psychological, 39
   Vocational, 39
Expectation, 180
Expert systems, 66

F

Fatigue, 129
   Mental, 130
   Muscle, 130
   Psychological, 130
Flexibility, 28, 118
Food and air cycles, 123
Foot Rest, 60
Force, 108
Formulas, 214
Functional abilities, 136
Functional capacity assessment, 103
   Categories, 106
   Current Issues, 105
   Factors in, 104
   Importance, 101
   Technology in, 104
Functional electric stimulation, 149, 174
   and LBP, 150
   Applications, 150
   Efficacy, 182
   Indications, 150
Functional restoration index, 144

H

Hand steadiness, 122
Herniated disk, 24, 40

Human
  Machine system, 4, 35
  Performance, 3, 101, 104
  Performance profile, 102, 106, 169
  Work, 127

I

Impairment, 11, 32, 105
Isoinertial, 129
Isokinetic, 128
Isometric, 111, 128
Isotonic, 128

J

Job
  Analysis, 56
  Classification, 28
  Demands, 7, 55
  Redesign, 58
  Simulation, 57, 152

K

Kinesiology, 120

L

Levers, 87
  First class, 88
  Mechanical advantage, 89
  Second class, 88
  Third class, 89
Lifting, 95
  Belt, 85
  Liftest, 137
  Maximum acceptable weight, 138
  Maximum dynamic weight, 137
Limitations, 106
Low back pain,
  and lifting, 31
  and occupation, 11, 28
  Acute, 31, 32
  Causes, 28, 42, 172
  Chronic, 31, 32
  Cost, 12
  Disability, 34
  Incidence, 10
  Management, 43
  Origin, 23
  Prevalence, 9
  Recurrence, 10
Lumbosacral angle, 17

M

Matching, 5, 6
Metabolism,
  Aerobic, 123
  Anaerobic, 123
  Basal rate, 124
  O_2 debt, 125
  O_2 uptake, 125
  Resting rate, 124
  Role of O_2, 125
Multipliers, 213
Muscle
  Action, 108
  Contraction, 109
  Fatigue, 130
  Force, 108
  Insertion, 20
  of the trunk, 20, 21, 25, 26
  Origin, 20

Muscle (*continued*)
  Paravertebral, 20
  Reeducation, 149, 183
  Spasms, 23
  Strength, 107
Muscular system, 19
Myofascial pain syndrome, 41
  Gluteal, 43
  Iliopsoas, 43
  Quadratus lumborum, 43
  Rectus abdominis, 43

N

Negative work, 129
Nerves, 19
NIOSH, 96

O

Obesity, 75
Occupational therapy, 39
Orthoranger, 120
Osteoporosis, 24, 26
Outcome, 140, 169

P

Pain, 8
  Acute, 32
  Centers, 43, 46
  Chronic, 32
  Cycle, 32
  Experience, 8
  Management, 35, 40, 43, 47
  Patient profile, 29
  Sensation, 8
Percentiles, 109
Physical measures, 106

Physical therapy, 38
Physician's evaluations, 37
Physiological measures, 123
Pre injury stage, 36
Positive work, 129
Post injury stage, 48
Post-rehabilitation stage, 52
Posture, 25, 28, 73, 165
  Adjustment, 80
  Awkward, 73, 77
  Dynamic 117
  Good, 74, 82
  Guidelines, 81
  Neutral, 79
  Planes of reference, 73, 75
  Restricted, 71
  Static, 117
Primary prevention, 35
Psychology, 39
Psychomotor abilities, 121

Q

Quadratus lumborum, 23, 43

R

Ranges of motion, 119
Reaction time, 121
Rehabilitation
  Approaches, 45
  Centers, 45
  Components, 50
  Goals of, 44, 49
  Medical, 40
  Multidisciplinary, 50
  Technological, 48
Restrictions, 106
Risk factors, 57

S

Screening, 103
Scoliosis, 24, 27
Secondary prevention, 35
Skeletal system, 14
Slipping and falling, 29
Spina bifida, 28
Spinal
  Column, 17
  Cord, 19
  Nerves, 19
  Shape, 18
  Stenosis, 24
  Hip mobility, 21
Spondylolisthesis, 24
Static, 93, 117, 128
Strength
  Dynamic, 117
  Grip, 115
  Instructions, 146
  Isokinetic, 117
  Measurement of, 144
  Positions, 112
  Procedures, 113
  Static, 114
Stress, 5, 6
Surgery, 47
SWAD, 66
Sway, 120

T

Tertiary prevention, 35
Tolerances, 136
Treatment, 44

V

Vertebral column, 14
Vertebrae
  Cervical, 16
  Lumbar, 16, 17
  Thoracic, 16, 17
VDT workplace, 62
Vocational evaluation, 39

W

Walking pace, 120
Weights, 137
Work
  Conditioning, 152
  Hardening, 153
  Injuries, 11
Workplace
  Analysis, 58, 178
  Design, 68, 71
  Dimensions, 67, 70